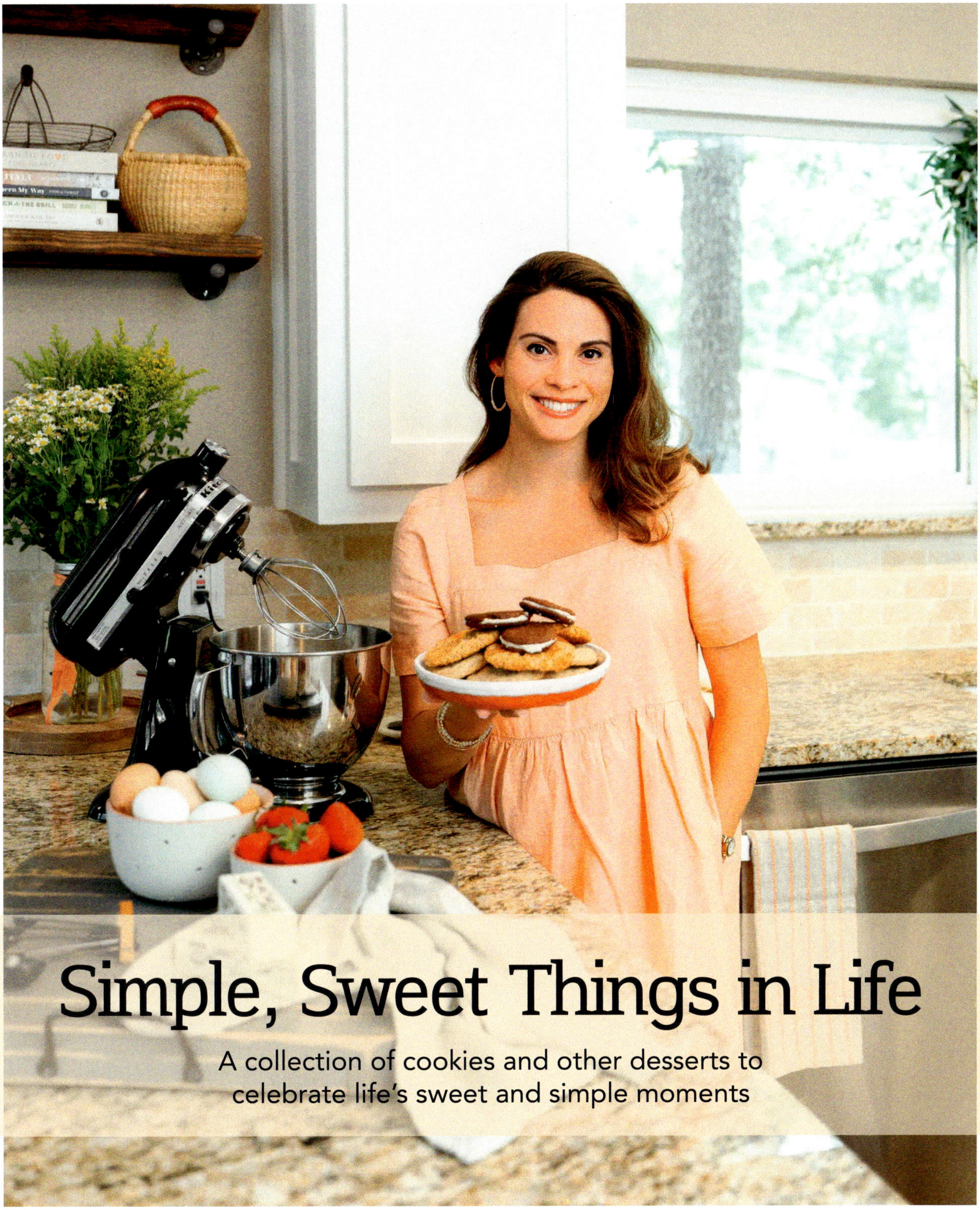

Simple, Sweet Things in Life

A collection of cookies and other desserts to celebrate life's sweet and simple moments

Stephanie Rackley RDN, LD

Published in the United States by Bacchus Publishing House,
an imprint of Legacy Print House, Houston, TX.
legacyprinthouse.com

Some recipes originally appeared on the author's website,
https://thehealthychew.org.

ISBN: 978-1-64943-084-7

Lifestyle and Front Cover Photography by Cortney Hostin
Book design by Vibha Jindal

Printed in the United States of America

First Printing Edition, 2021

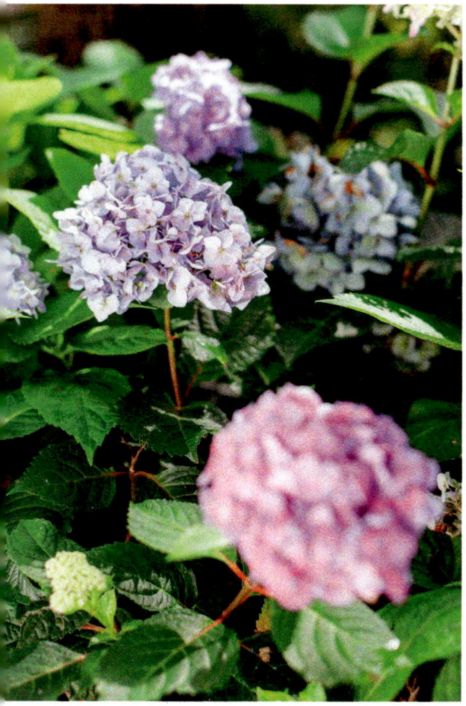

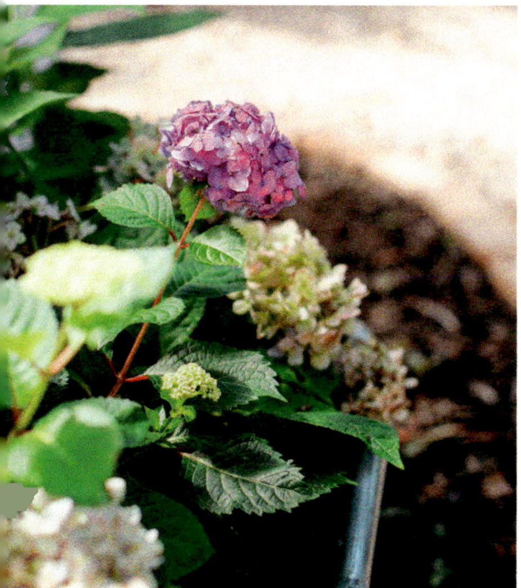

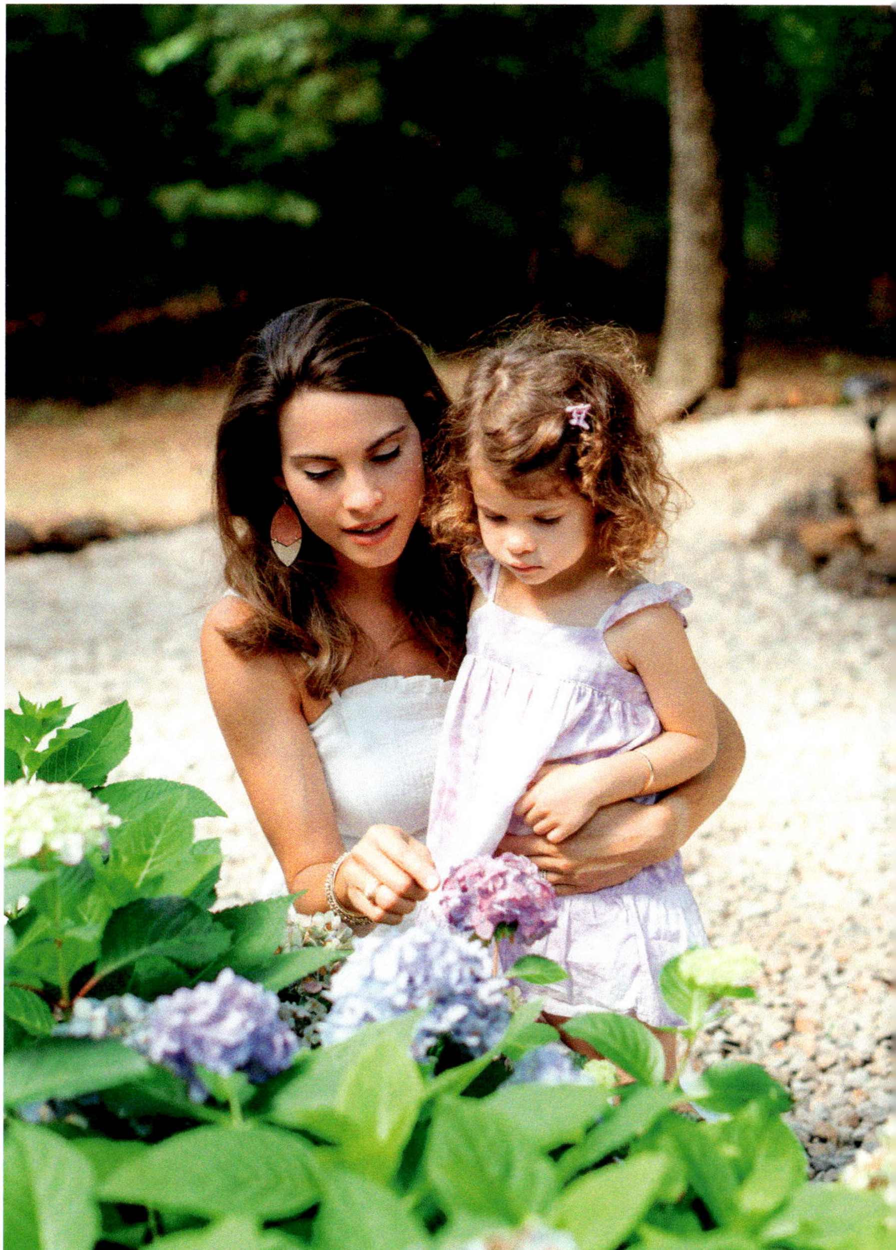

Table of Contents

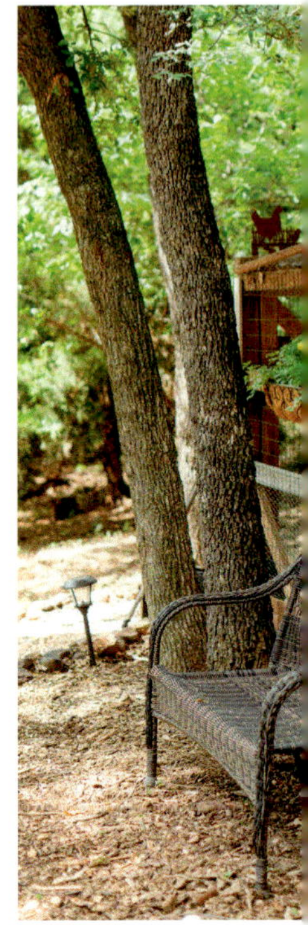

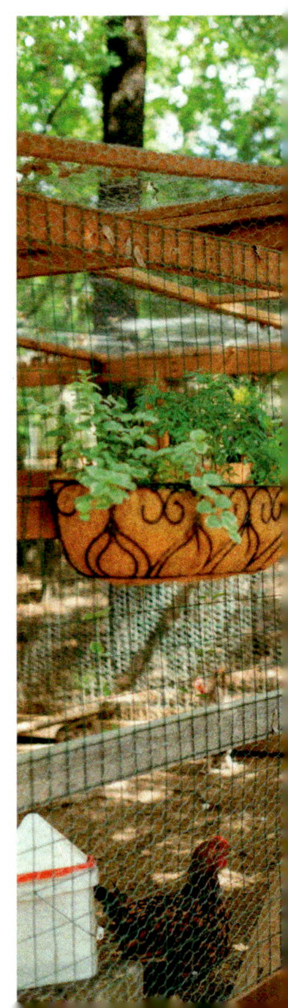

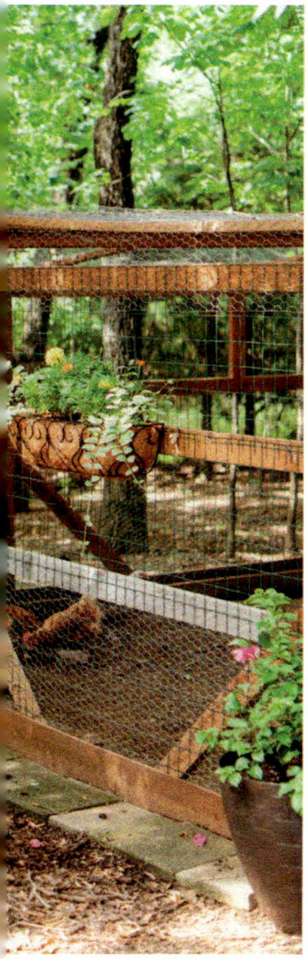

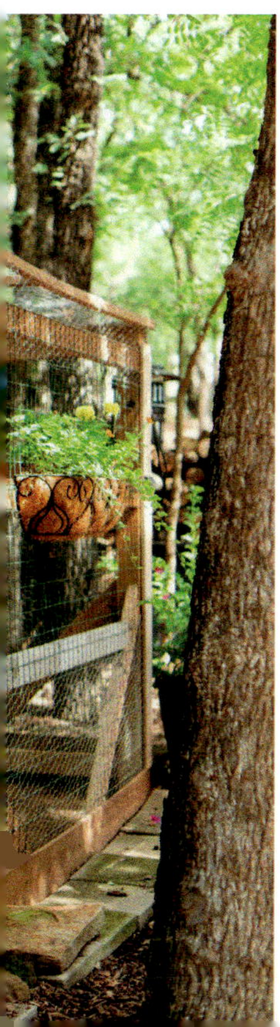

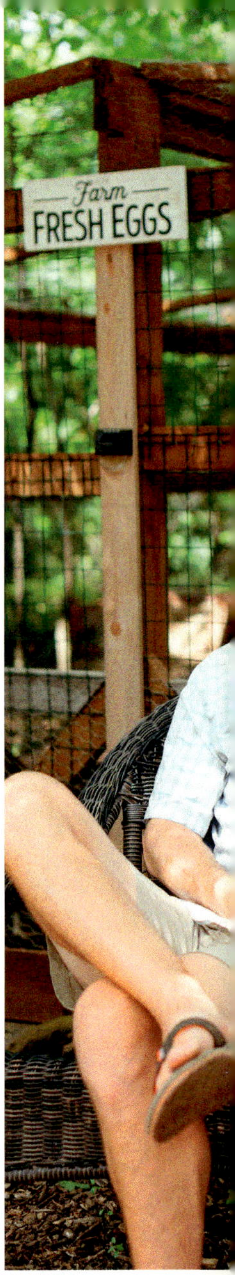
Farm
FRESH EGGS

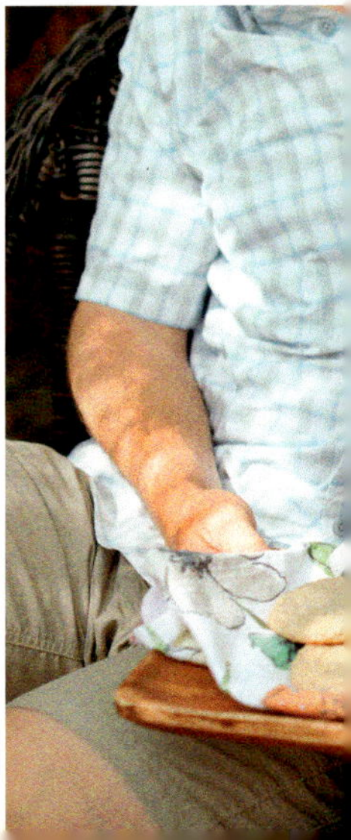

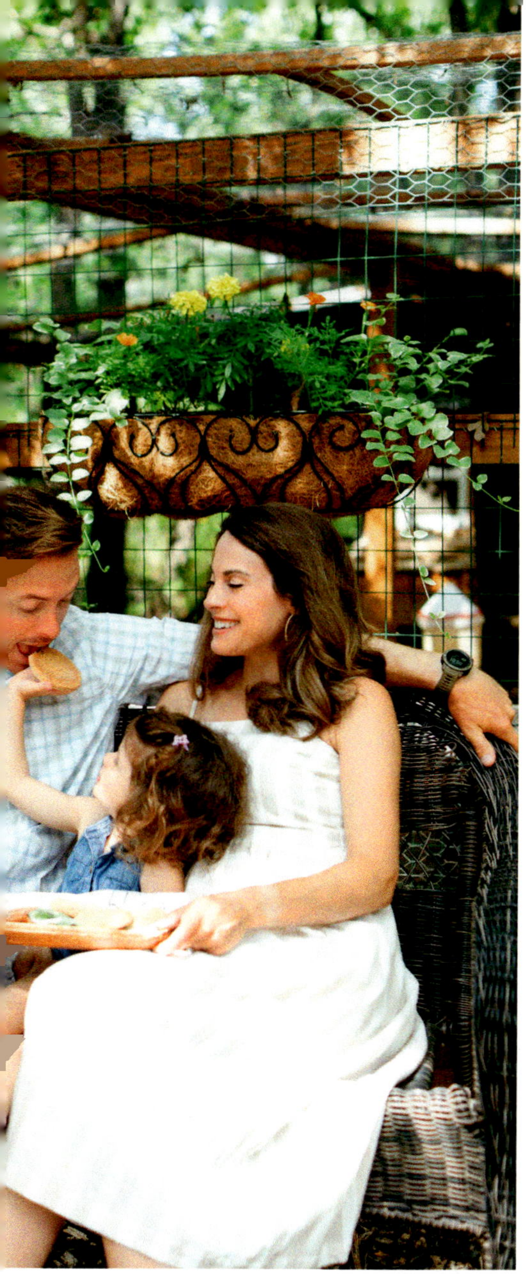
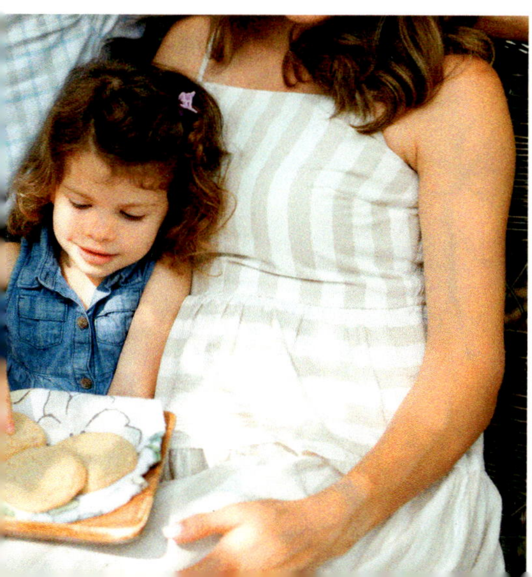
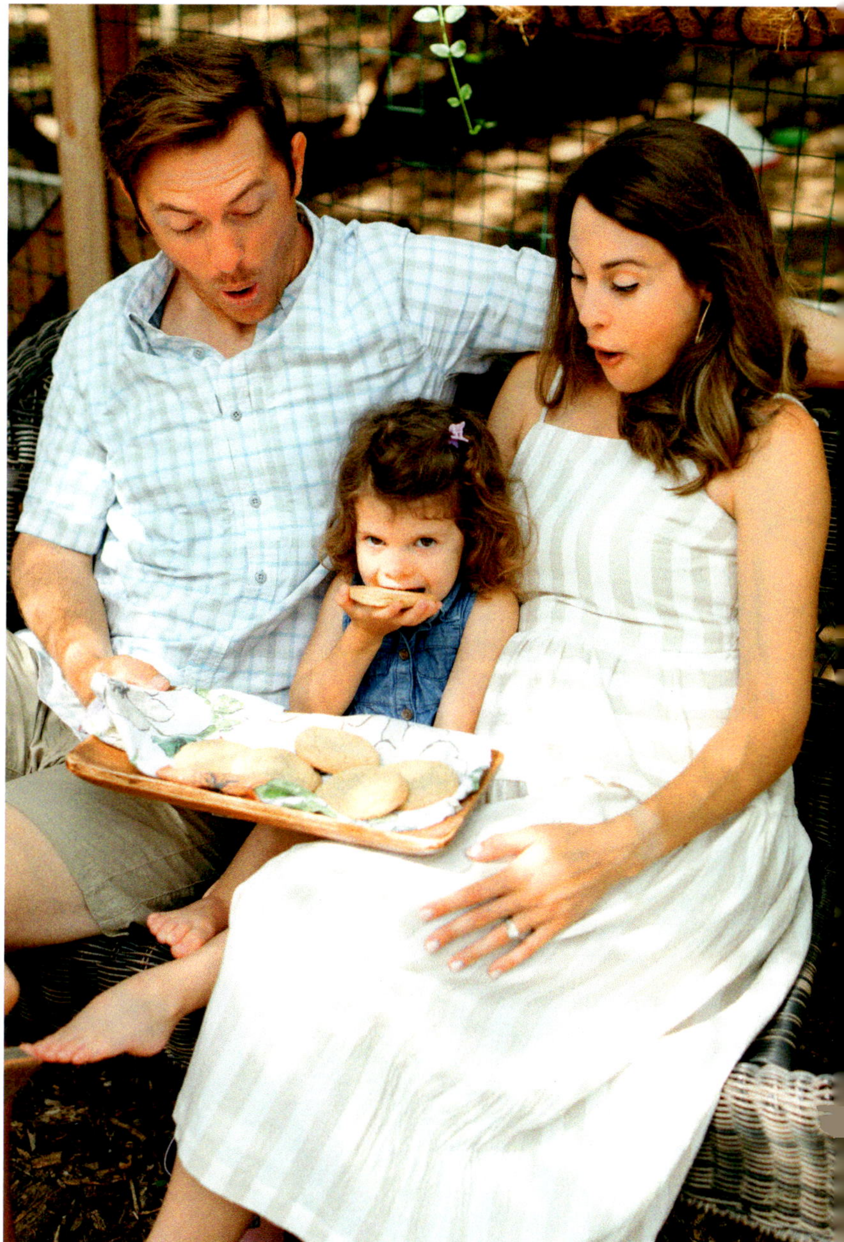

Allergy Guide

Dairy Free

Sugar Free

Gluten Free

Egg Free

Nut Free

Soy Free

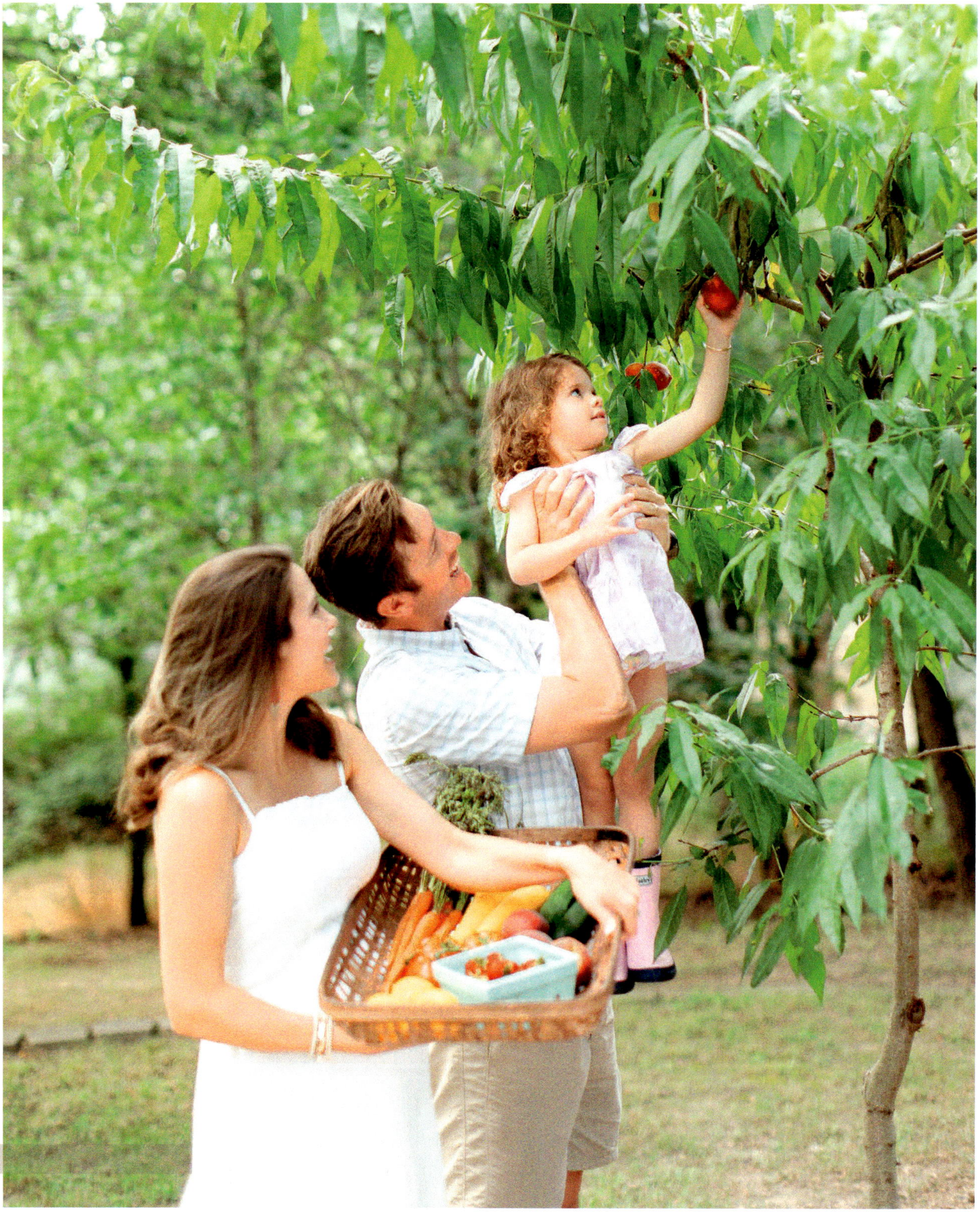

Thank You

Thank you to my sweet, yet incredibly honest husband, Justin, for taste-testing every single recipe that went into this book. Your support from the very beginning of our marriage has not only led me to pursue my passion in the kitchen but also given me drive and mountainous motivation.

Thank you to my sweet family, both Mimi & LFD and Nana & Tata for the unmeasurable amount of support, weekly taste-testings, and honest opinions that gave me room to grow and dream bigger than before.

Thank you to my sweet Emmie girl. I hope you hold onto these memories and look back on this book with joy & happiness.

To all of you who hold a copy of this cookbook in your hands, thank you for following along on this amazing journey. This book truly would not have happened without so many of you asking for it, pleading for it, and wanting my recipes to have a place in your home and on your table.

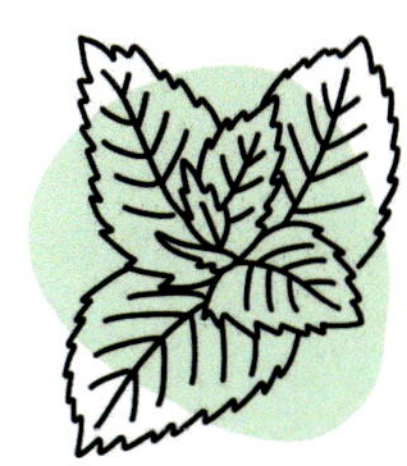

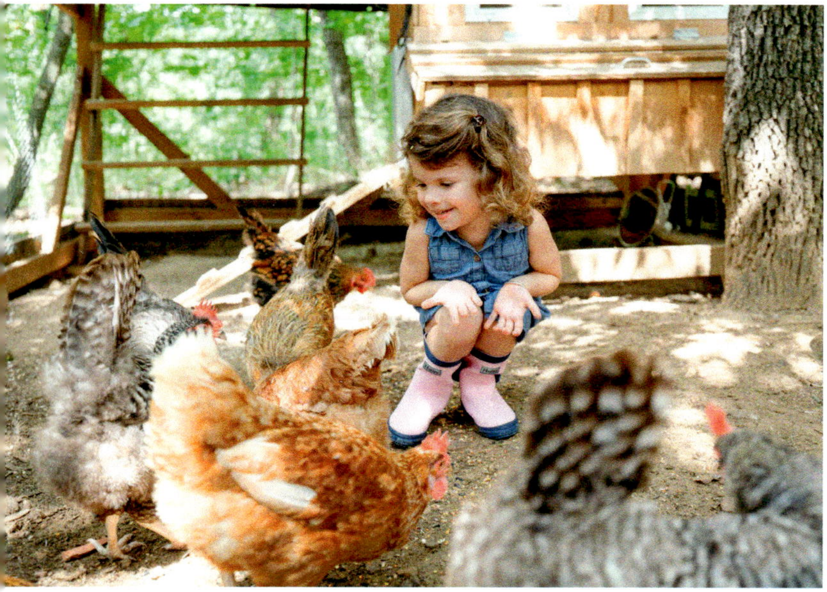

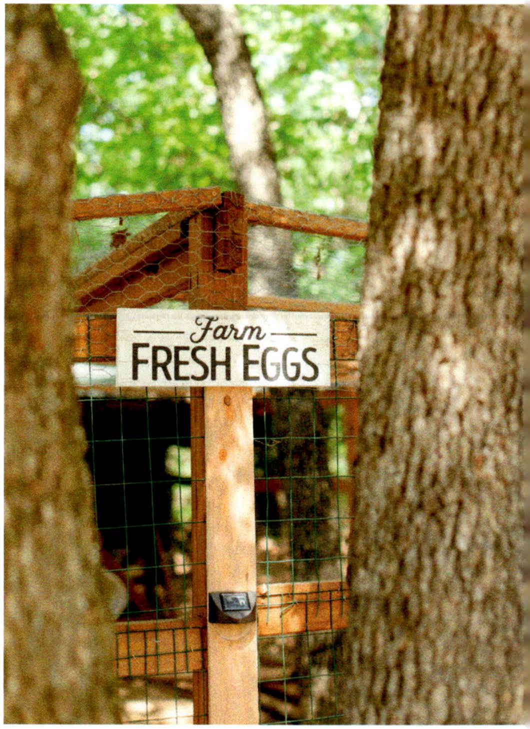
Farm
FRESH EGGS

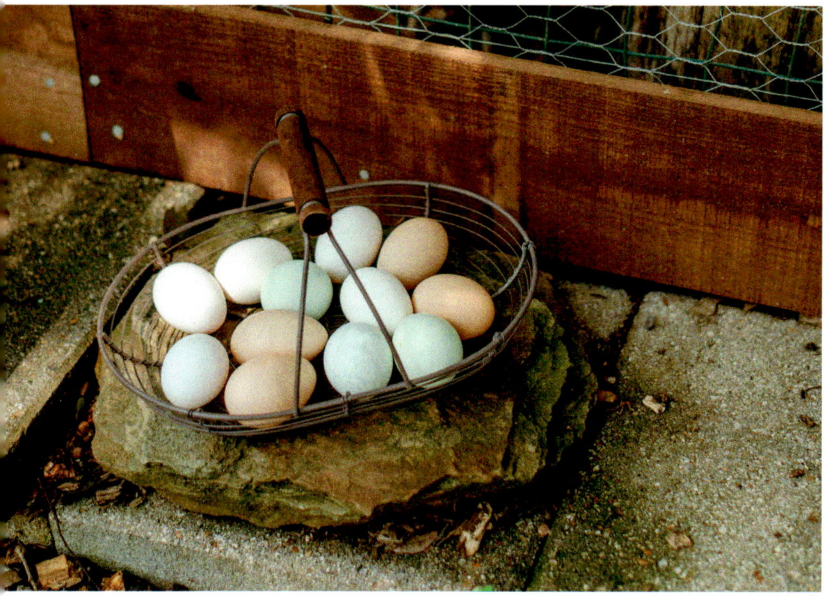

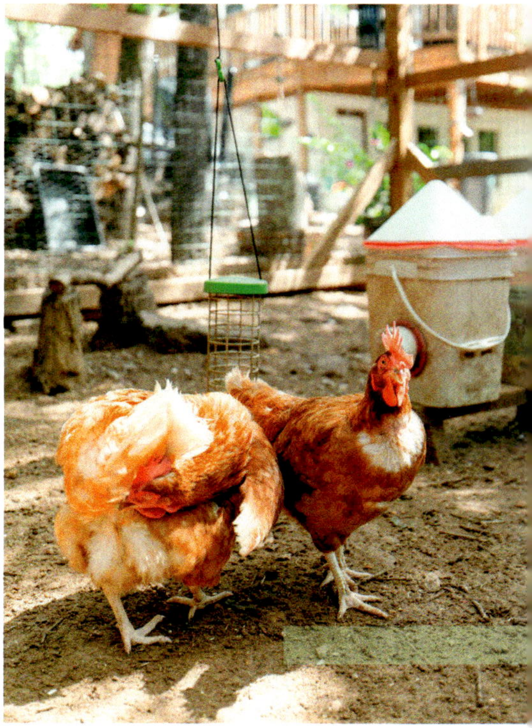

Life's Simple, Sweet Things

Summer rainstorms • Baby tummy kicks • Toddler hands reaching up for a hug • *Hearing the words "I love you" for the first time* • Freshly picked strawberries • Ripe peach juice dripping down your chin • *Homemade dessert on a Sunday evening* • Family gatherings around the dinner table • Rolling down the windows • A summer's golden sunset • A good conversation with an old friend • Picking tulips • Fresh flowers in the kitchen • *The smell of freshly baked cookies* • Baking with butter • Slow Sunday evenings on the back patio • Hearing your baby's belly laugh for the first time • Iced coffee on a hot summer day • The smell of pumpkin spice on a chilly fall day *Homemade buttermilk biscuits* • Freshly mowed grass • Colorful spring hydrangeas • Waking up early to see the sunrise • Sweet newborn baby smell • *A day spent on the lake* • Sun-kissed shoulders • Ice-cold lemonade from the neighborhood kids • *Farm fresh eggs* • Freshly-picked fragrant herbs • Toddlers swinging on rope swings • Rain boots splashing in puddles • Roasting s'mores on a chilly fall evening • *A fresh haul from the local farmers market* • Sandy beach toes and salty kisses • Fresh-squeezed orange juice for breakfast • A relaxing cup of chamomile tea before bedtime • *Gifting homemade Christmas cookies* • Picking peaches in the summer • Fresh Banana bread baking in the kitchen • Drinking coffee on the front porch steps • Running through the sprinklers as a child • *A barefoot walk on the beach* • Taking the family camping in the fall • Crisp fall mornings • Freshly fallen snow in the wintertime • *Freshly baked cookies and a cold glass of milk* • Rocking chairs on the back porch

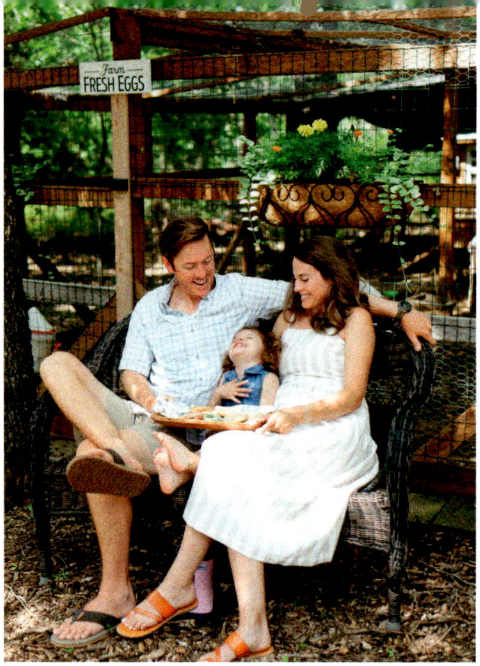

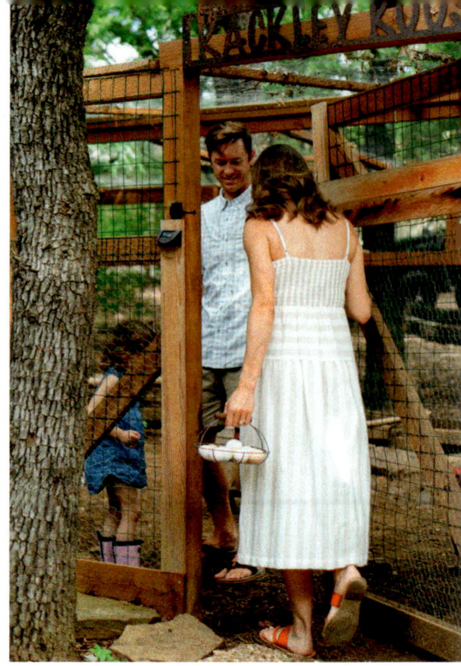

A Note from the Author

Why is this book specially curated for you?

A little about my history in the food and nutrition world - This dessert cookbook has been nothing short of a crazy personal journey for me. When just beginning on this project, collecting recipes and deciding how to create such a book, I was diagnosed with Hashimoto's Thyroiditis disease.

In the same week of learning about this diagnosis, I found out I was pregnant with our second child. I was taken aback by this diagnosis, since I have to watch everything that I put on my plate. I've always lived a balanced lifestyle, one that includes plenty of fibrous vegetables and plant-based nutrients. I have proudly raised my family on scratch-made meals, and I've made it my mission in life to share my nutrition knowledge with the public.

First and foremost, I am a Registered and Licensed Dietitian who has experienced a fair share of food sensitivities. For the last ten years, my body has been sensitive to soy-based foods and products. Creating a lifestyle diet around this obstacle has been a blessing in disguise and ultimately gave way to my passion for cooking and baking from scratch. After being diagnosed with Hashimoto's Thyroiditis, my food sensitivities continued to expand and get worse. For months I had to avoid gluten, eggs, soy, dairy, caffeine, and alcohol. These foods acted as triggers for my autoimmune disease.

As I embarked on creating a dessert cookbook, I found a new challenge of creating delicious sweet treats with food triggers in mind. Having to go through this elimination diet and pull common allergens out of my daily diet, I was continually reminded of how many people suffer from food allergies on a daily basis. So, not only did I want to create a beautiful story with our beloved family dessert recipes, but I wanted to create a cookbook that anybody could pick up and enjoy.

Regardless of your food allergies, regardless of your family's necessary modifications, regardless of your current health situation, there is something for everybody in this cookbook. I've made sure to include options that are free from gluten, dairy, nuts, eggs, peanuts and soy. Other recipes that contain no added sugar. Even a few are low-glycemic recipes. For me, having these options readily available was especially important because I understand how frustrating it can be to have limited food options.. I understand the need for creating such a book, and I wanted to be the one who shares it with you.

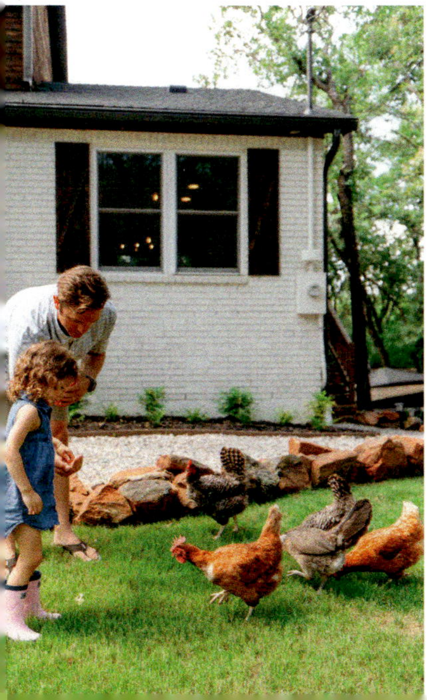

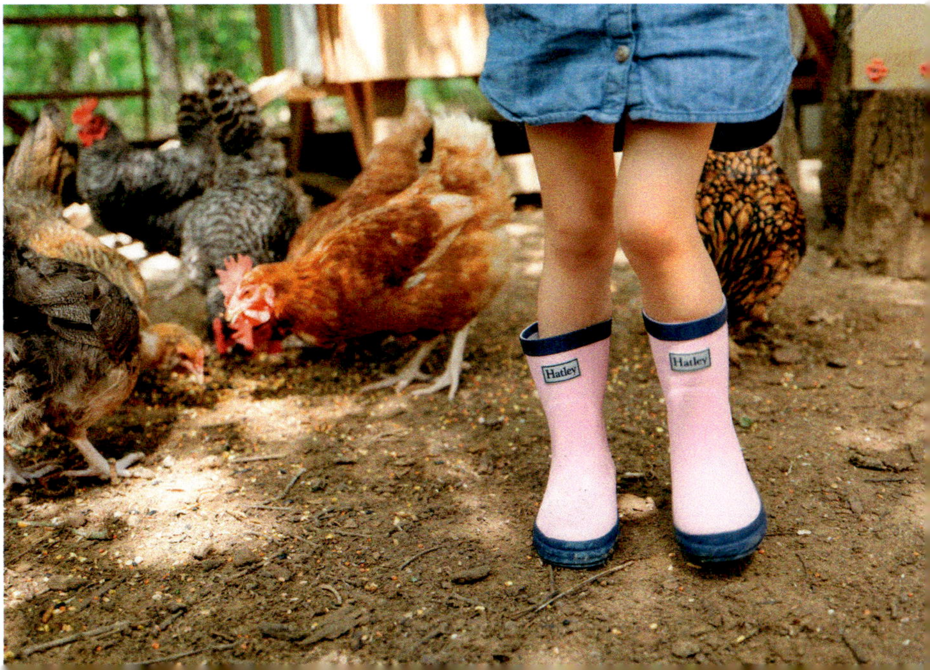

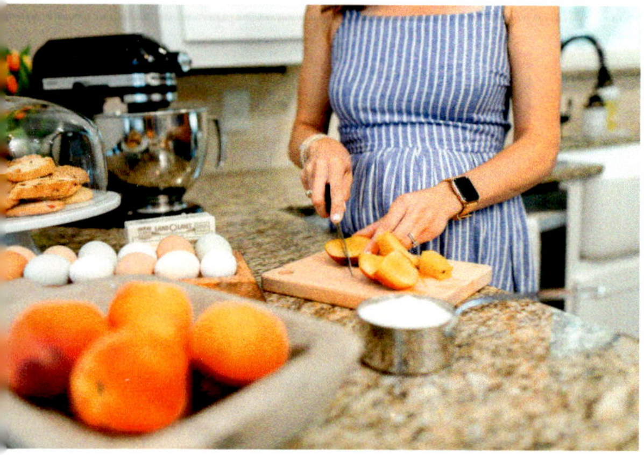

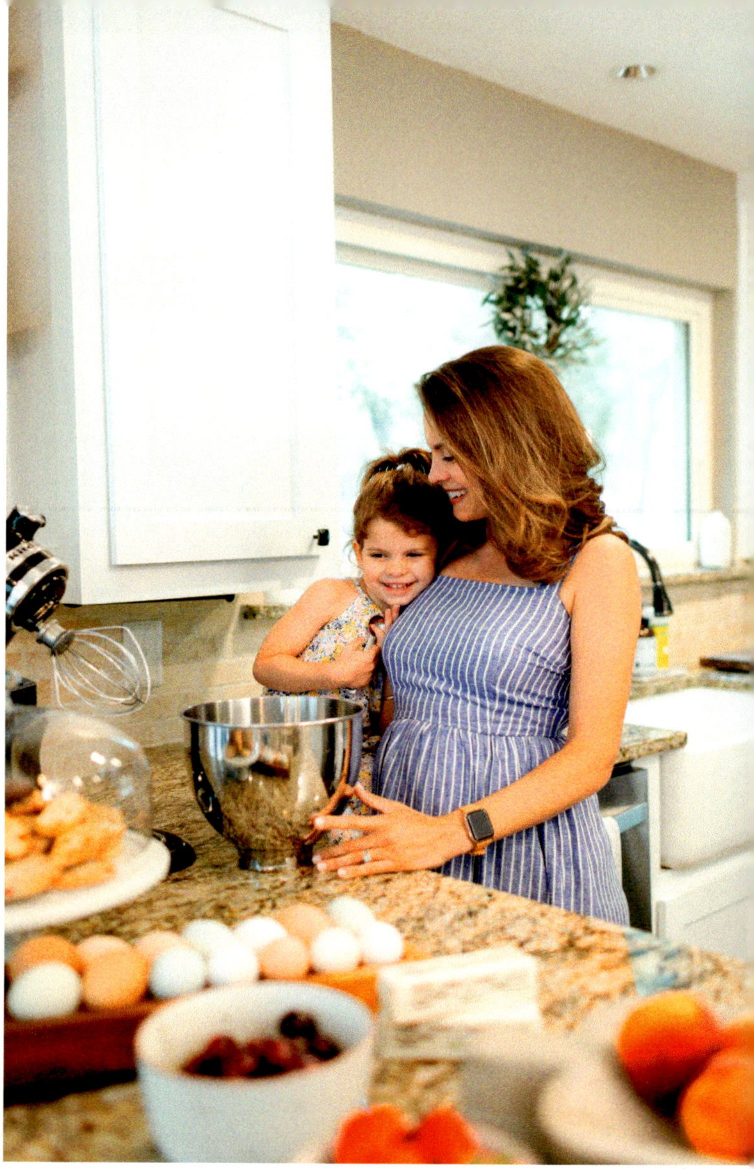

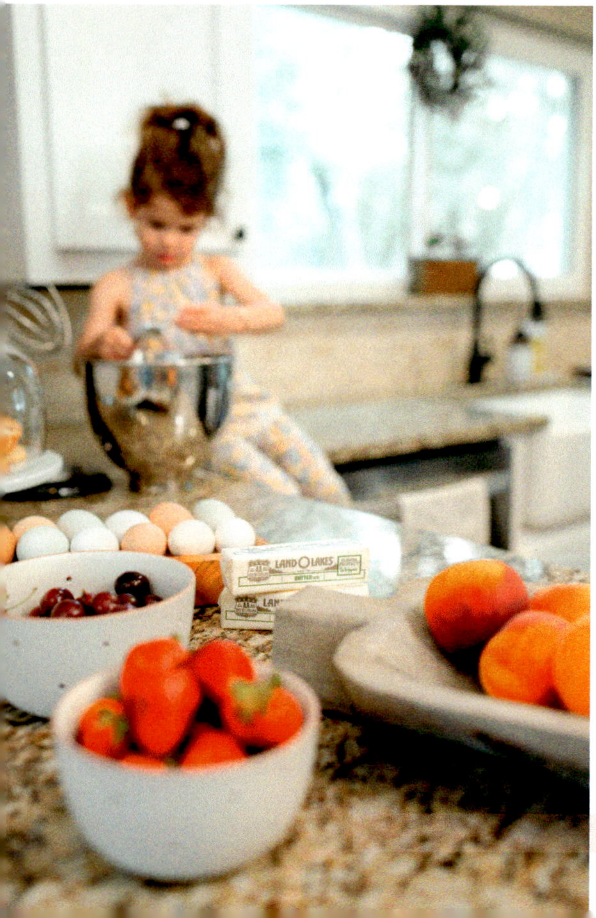
LAND O LAKES

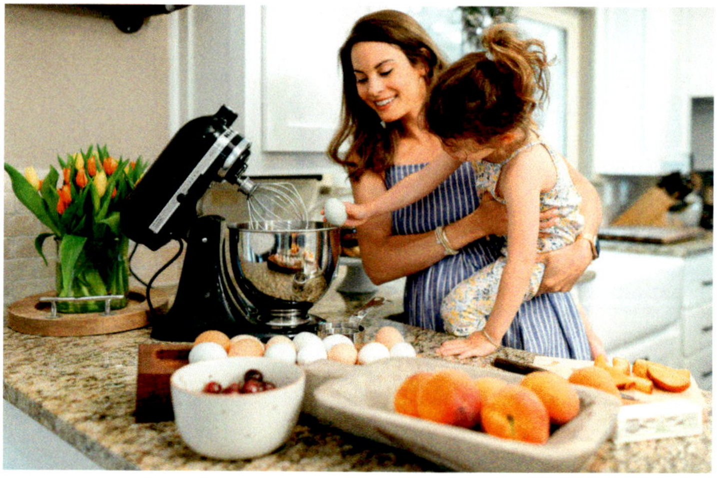

Introduction

This cookbook has been a long time coming, and I am beyond words in describing how much it means to me that you have decided to pick it up and indulge in the *Simple, Sweet Things in Life.* When beginning of the journey of writing this book, I knew I wanted to create something more than just a collection of recipes. Yes, these recipes are some of my family's most loved and talked about desserts that I am honored to be sharing. However I also wanted to share with you how we grew to love them. To me, food is personal and there's nothing more personal than dessert. Dessert has stories to be told, has all different faces and personalities, has all different seasons, and has all different ways of being enjoyed - even in the simplest of ways. Sometimes the sweetest things in life are the simplest, like when a plain bowl of vanilla ice cream gets topped off with fresh-picked summer berries. I've always enjoyed viewing life with a simplistic view to create beauty and serenity wherever I go. Enjoying the simple moments throughout the day and not rushing through my cup of hot tea in the mornings. Although I enjoy simplifying our home, lifestyle, and meals, I still believe in dessert like an old fashioned mantra. I believe dessert is what brings people together. It's what keeps the conversation going at the table. And most importantly it creates a sense of home. This is ultimately what I hope to be sharing with you - my home. I've opened my front door and let you come inside. Please come in and stay a while as I take you on a journey through our simplest, sweetest things in life.

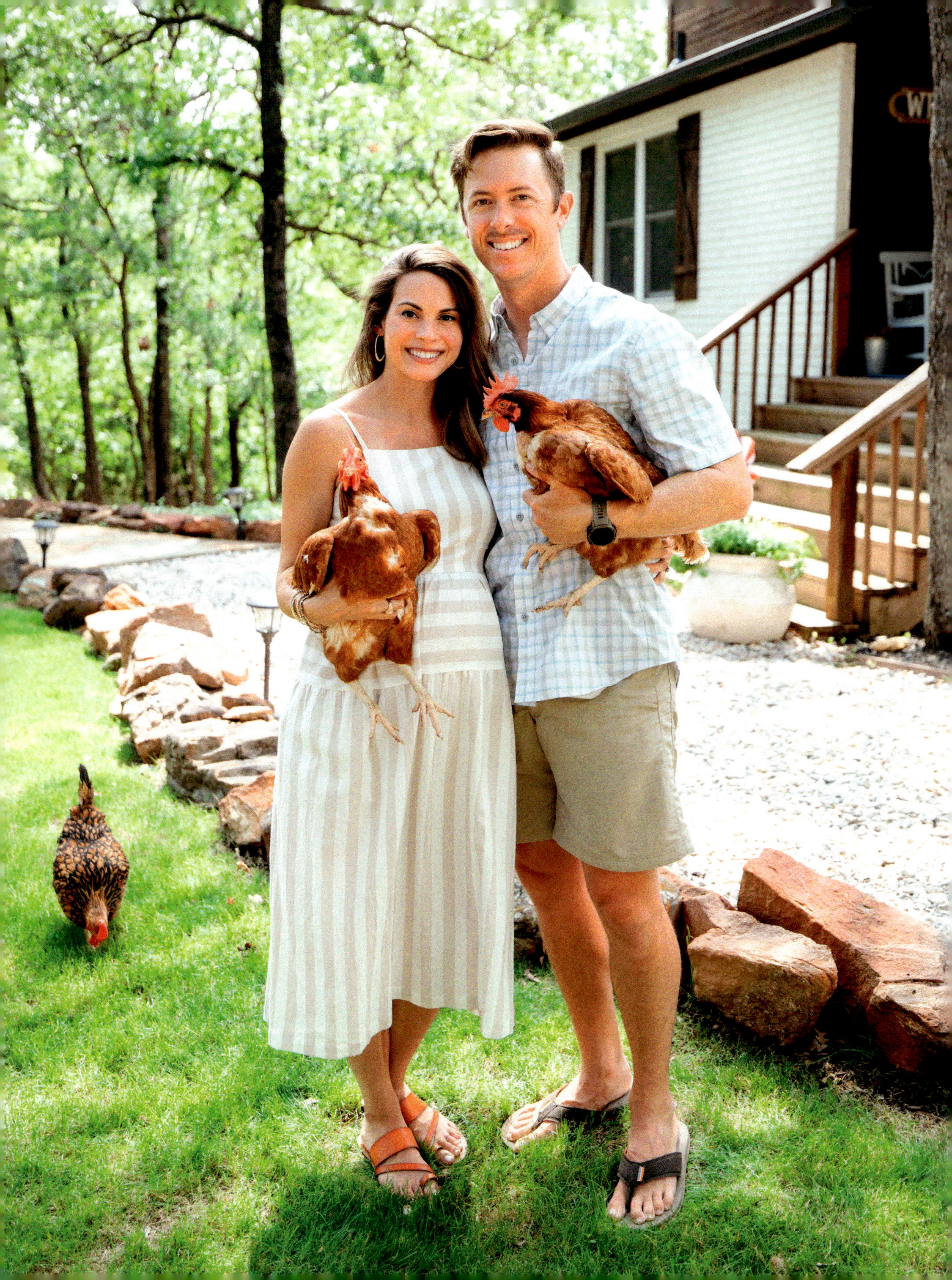

Kitchen Conversions

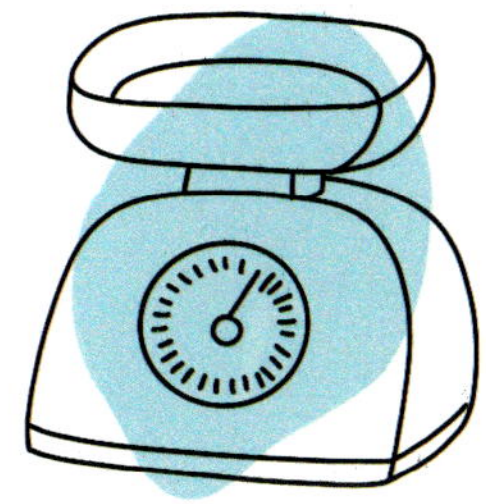

DRY VOLUME		
	1/8 teaspoon	1 pinch
	3 teaspoons	1 tablespoon
	1/8 cup	2 tablespoons
	1/4 cup	4 tablespoons
	1/2 cup	8 tablespoons
	3/4 cup	12 tablespoons
	1 cup	16 tablespoons
	1 pound	16 ounces

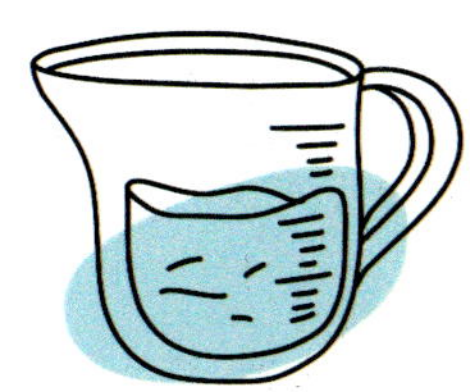

LIQUID VOLUME			
	8 fluid ounces	1 cup	
	1/2 pint	1 cup	
	1 pint	2 cups	
	1 quart	2 pints	4 cups
	1 gallon	4 quarts	16 cups

Tools of the Trade

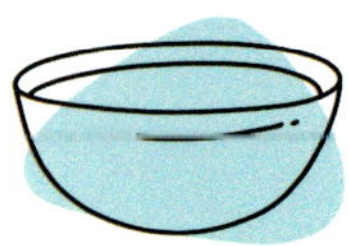

Mixing Bowls

Any mixing bowl will do, but a nice, sturdy bowl that is dishwasher safe will last many years to come. Multiple sizes will come in handy for whatever you want to throw together.

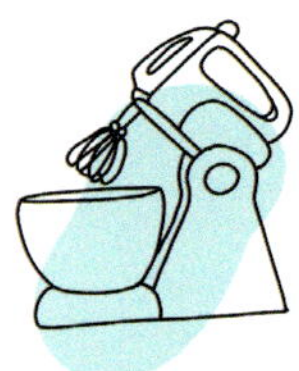

Stand Mixer

A stand mixer comes with several different mixing attachments that make life in the kitchen so much easier. If cared for properly, it will last a lifetime.

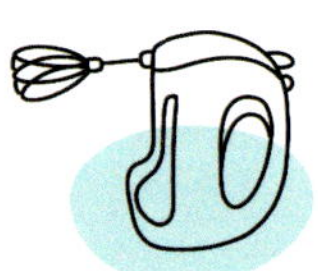

Hand Mixer

Hand mixers are perfect for mixing up small batches of whipped cream or making a delicious merengue without pulling out your heavy stand mixer.

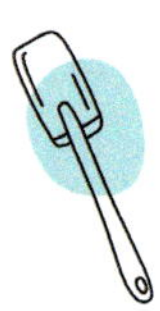

Silicone Spatula

Perfect for scraping out the sides of your mixing bowls, silicone spatulas come in different sizes that every kitchen needs.

Flat Spatula

You'll use a flat spatula for transferring your treats from the baking sheet to the cooling rack.

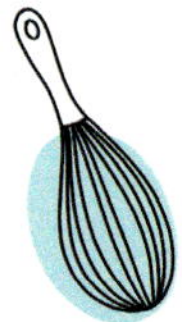

Whisk

Whether you choose stainless steel or silicone, a good whisk can have many uses in your kitchen.

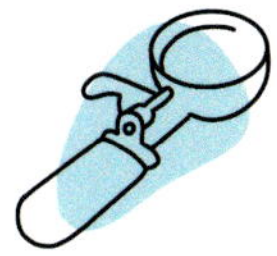

Scoops #100 (2 teaspoons) and #40 (2 tablespoons)

I use these two different size scoops to make the perfect size cookies. Although not an exact equivalent, a Scoop #100 is very close to 2 teaspoons or a 1-inch cookie ball, and a Scoop #40 is very close to 2 tablespoons or a 1 ½ inches cookie ball.

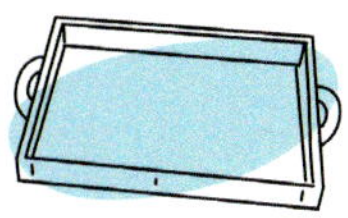

Baking Sheets

Quality baking sheets will last many, many years if cared for properly. Hand washing is recommended.

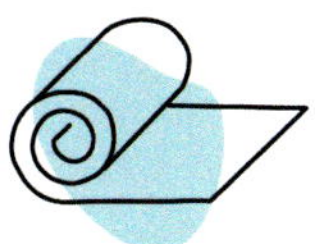

Parchment Paper

To save yourself some cleanup time, line baking sheets with parchment paper.

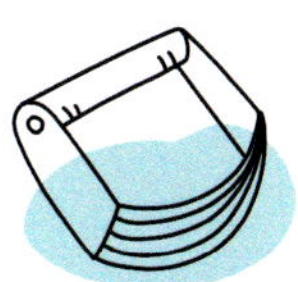

Pastry Cutter

Also called a dough cutter, this gadget cuts through flour and cold butter when making biscuits, scones, and other pastries. Make sure to find one that feels comfortable in your hand.

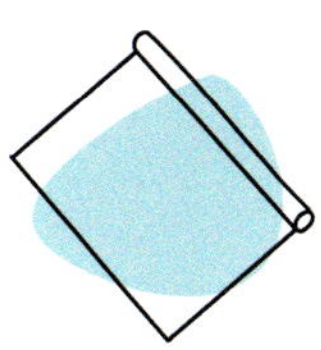

Pastry Scraper

A good pastry scraper will help you gently lift delicate pastries from your working space, but it can also double as a slicer when baking up a delicious batch of cinnamon rolls.

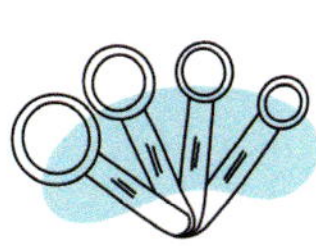

Measuring Spoons

You can find measuring spoons just about anywhere, as plain or as decorative as you want. Use what inspires you!

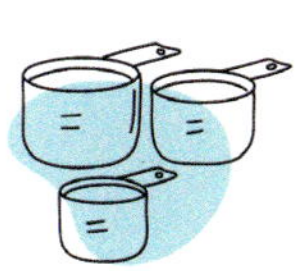

Measuring Cups

Just like measuring spoons, the cups you use should be durable and a tool that feels comfortable in your hand.

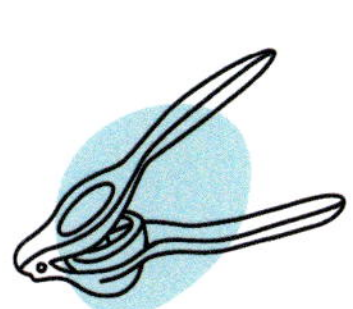

Lemon Juicer

Lemon juicers come in several varieties, but a hand-held juicer is easy to store and a quick way to juice your lemons.

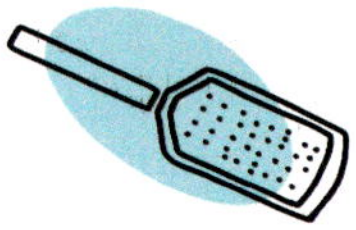

Lemon Zester

A lemon zester is another tool you can find in different styles. The style shown here is a microplane grater.

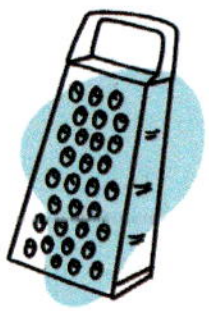

Grater

The grater is a kitchen staple. The different sizes can be used for anything from zesting lemons to grating cheese.

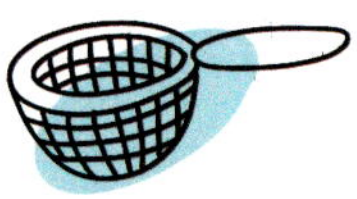

Sifter/Small Strainer AKA Sieve

A sieve will be your best friend when it comes to sifting flour and other ingredients. Taking the quick, extra step to sift your flour will help your recipes turn out fluffier.

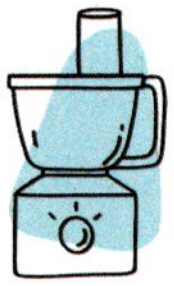

Food Processor

A food processor is a wonderful gadget that helps cut down on chopping time. From creating large chunks to puree, a food processor can do it all.

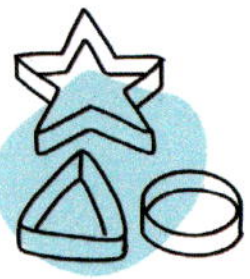

Large Biscuit/Cookie Cutter

When you think of biscuits, you generally imagine round, fluffy delicacies. Don't be afraid to get creative and use different shapes for your pastries!

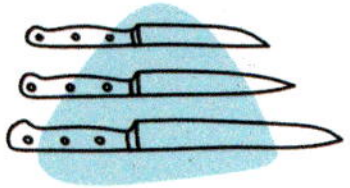

Quality Knives

Quality knives are another kitchen staple! The higher the quality, the longer they will last. I recommend you to wash your knives by hand.

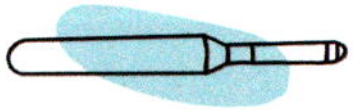

Icing Spatula

The icing spatula is specially designed to add icing to your desserts. Spreading icing is much easier when using this tool.

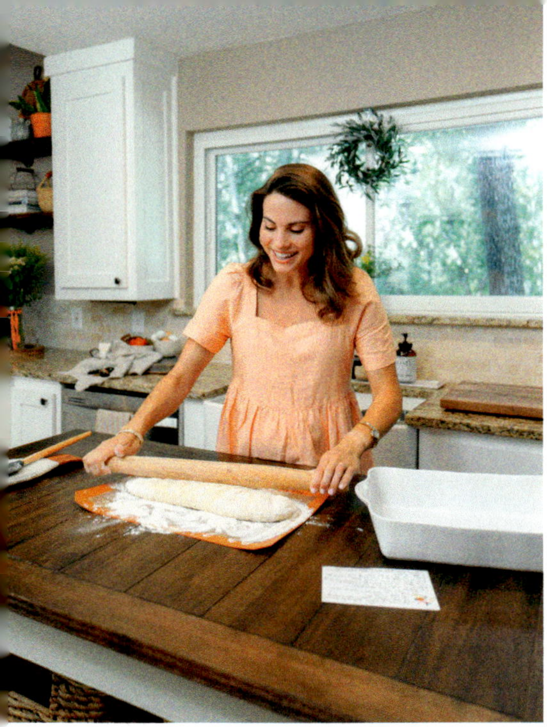

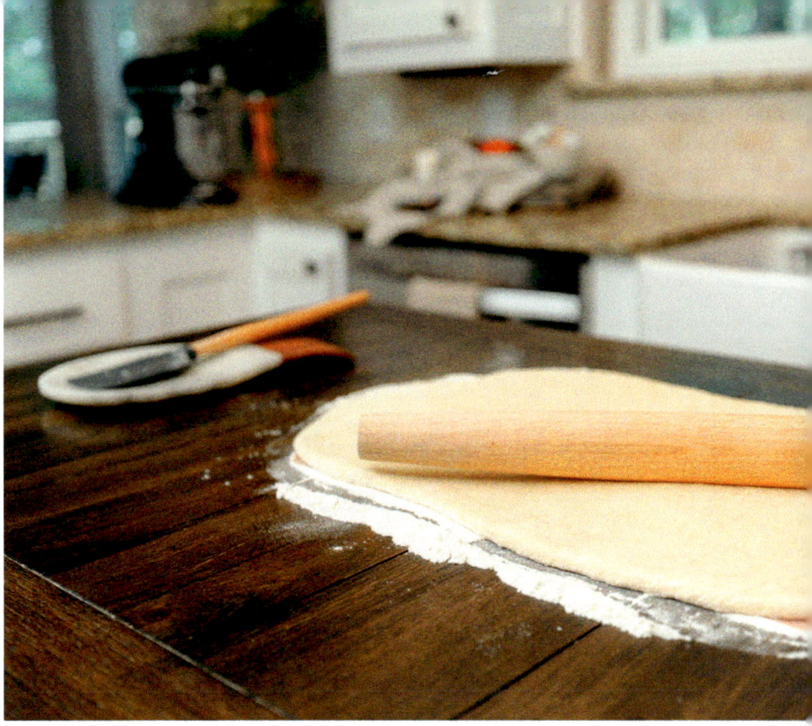

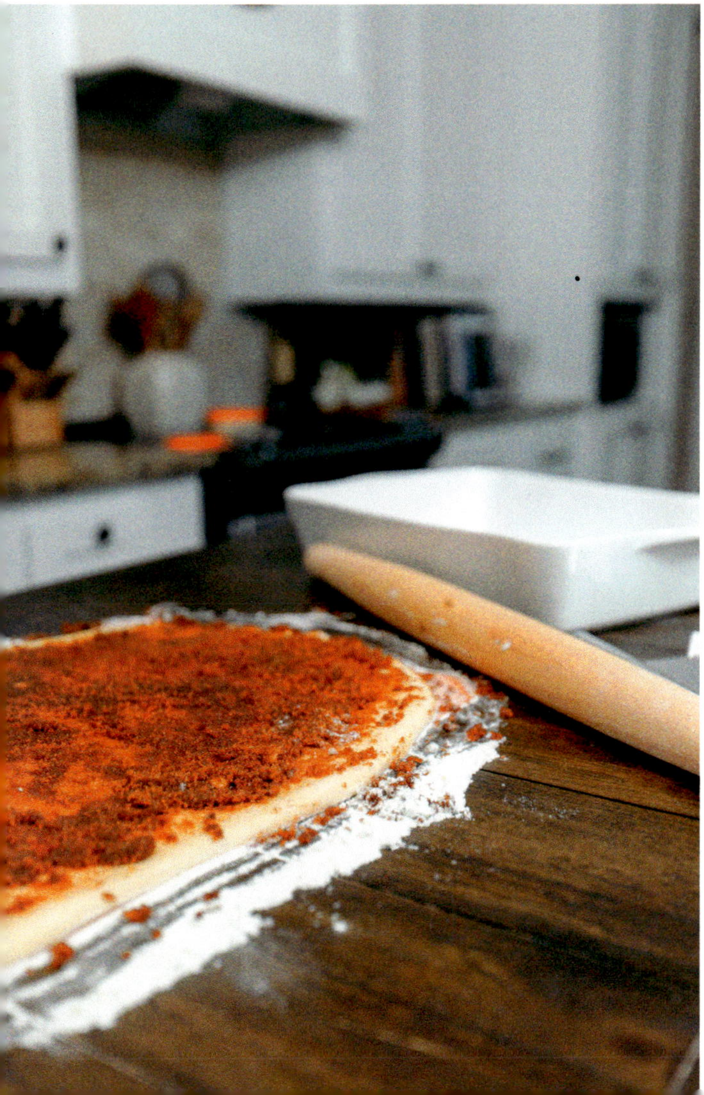

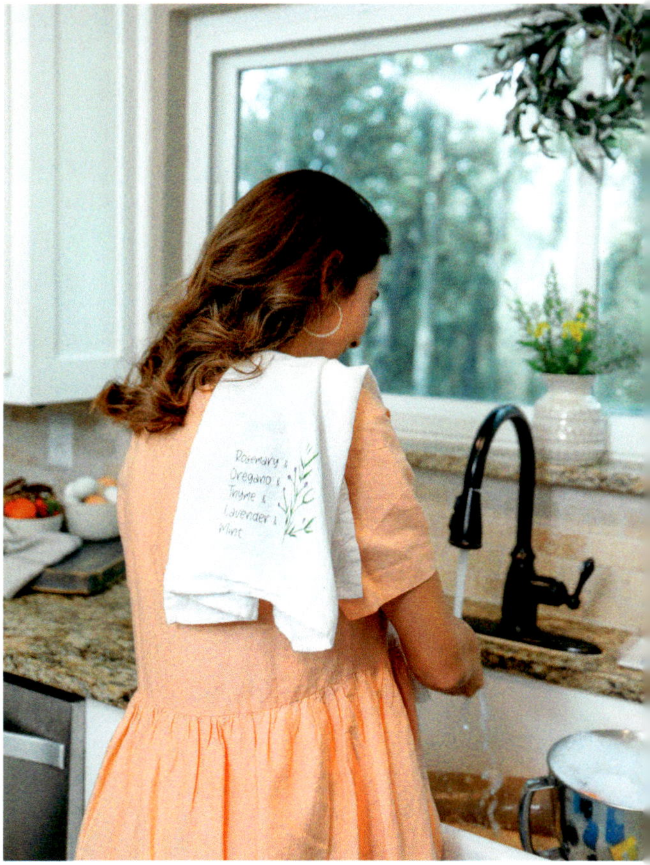
Rosemary &
Oregano &
Thyme &
Lavender &
Mint

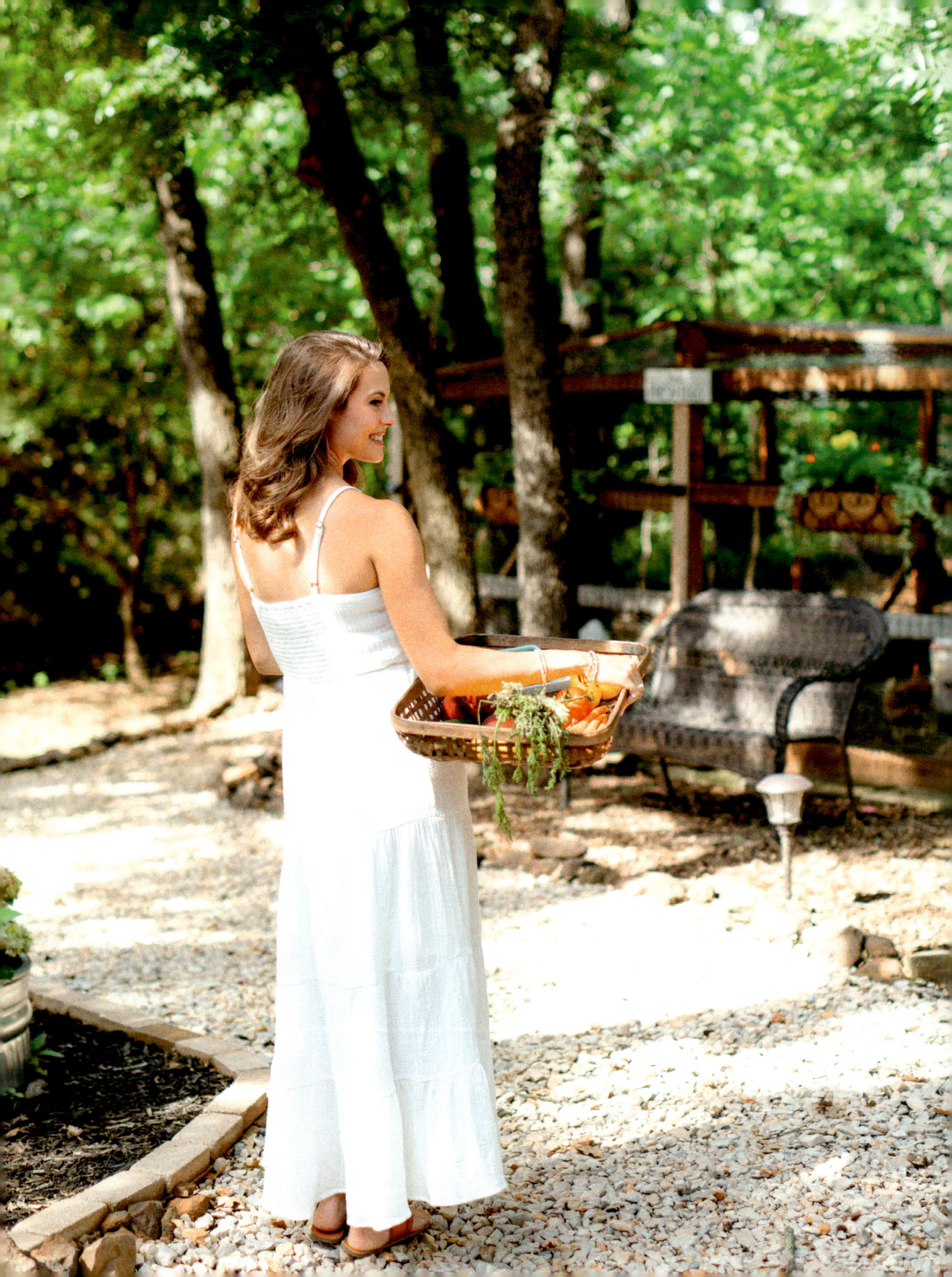

Sweet Picks from the Garden

- Twice Baked Apple Fritters
- Fresh Squeezed Orange Cranberry Cookies
- Carrot Zucchini Muffin Cookies
- Blueberry Sour Cream Cookies *(Nana's Pick)*
- Banana Bread Walnut Cookies *(Tata's Pick)*
- Pucker Up Lemon Sugar Cookies
- Summertime Strawberry Scone Cookies
- Get Figgy With It-Breakfast Biscotti
- Decadent Raspberry Cream Cheese Danish Cookies
- Mini Peach Pie Cookie Cups

Fruit & Vegetable Classification

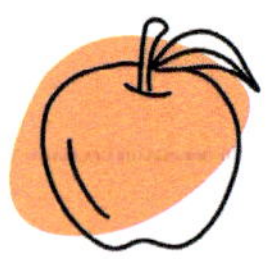

Apple: a-p-l
Contains a thin layer of edible skin on the outside with a crisp texture on the inside. Apples contain seeds in their cores and come in many different colors. Apples contain antioxidants, vitamins, dietary fiber, and may help to reduce the risk of cancer, obesity, heart disease, and diabetes.

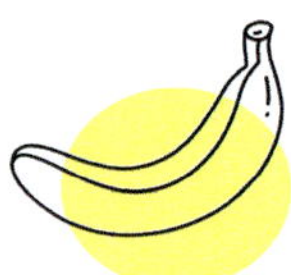

Banana: Buh-na-nuh
Contains a thick inedible peel that must be stripped in order to get to the fruit inside. Bananas are mainly yellow in color.
Bananas are rich in potassium, which can help to lower blood pressure. They also contain fiber, folate, and antioxidants such as vitamin C.

Blueberry: Bloo-beh-ree
Small and round in shape, blueberries have a deep, rich, blue color.They are sweet yet slightly tart to the taste.
Blueberries are rich in antioxidants such as anthocyanin. They also contain vitamin C, vitamin K, iron, calcium, magnesium, zinc, folate and fiber.

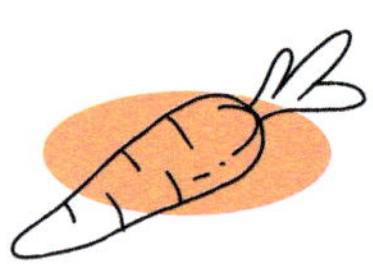

Carrot: Keh-ruht
Considered a root vegetable, carrots have a bright orange color and a firm, crisp skin.
Excellent source of alpha and beta-carotene, lutein, and zeaxanthin.

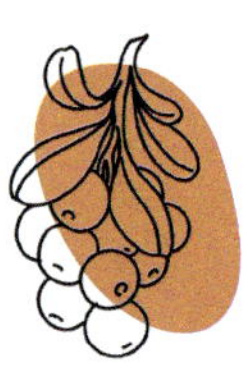

Cranberry: Kran-beh-ree
Small and slightly oblong in shape, cranberries contain a deeply rich red color and are tart to the taste.
Good source of fiber and vitamin C. Cranberries are known to have additional benefits such as an antimicrobial effect.

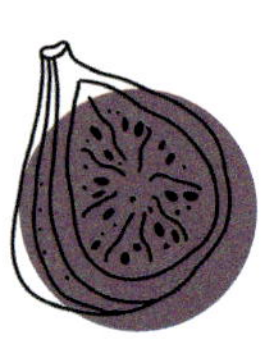

Fig: Fig
The edible fruit grown from a ficus carica tree, figs are pear shaped and contain hundreds of seeds inside.
Great source of fiber, magnesium, and manganese. Dried figs also contain calcium and iron.

Lemon: Leh-muhn

Bright yellow in color, this football shaped fruit is sour to the taste. Both the juice and the skin are used in baking.
Rich in vitamin C and fiber, lemons aid in heart and digestive health.

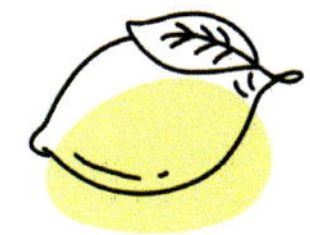

Orange: Aw-ruhnj

Orange in color and round in shape, both the skin and juice are used in baking. Navel oranges are most common.
Great source of vitamin C. Contains folate and potassium as well.

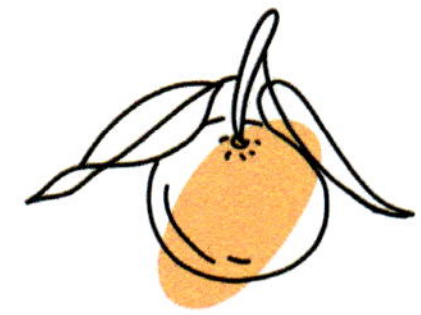

Peach: Peech

Considered a stone fruit, peaches are sweet and ripe during the summer months. They contain an edible furry skin and a large pit inside.
Rich in vitamin C and other antioxidants, peaches help to reduce inflammation and oxidative stress in the body.

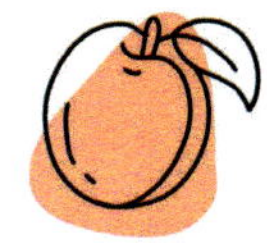

Raspberry: Raz-beh-ree

These small delicate berries that contain visible seeds on the outside are deeply red and contain a sweetly tart taste.
A great source of fiber, manganese, vitamin C, and vitamin K.

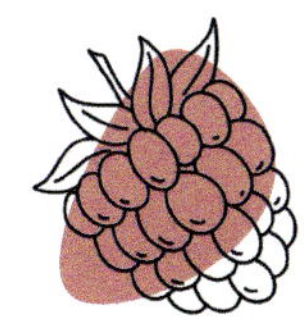

Strawberry: Straa-beh-ree

Not technically a berry, the strawberry is a heart-shaped fruit containing seed achenes on the outside. Red in color and sweet to the taste, strawberries ripen in the early spring.
Great source of vitamin C. Also contains anthocyanin, which creates the red color. Strawberries boost antioxidant levels in the blood. Eating a diet rich in strawberries is known to have health benefits such as reducing risk for heart disease and cognitive decline.

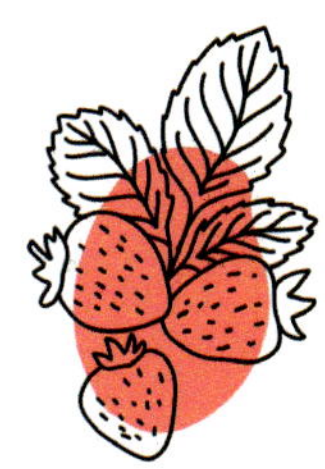

Zucchini: Zoo-kee-nee

Easy to grow in a home garden, zucchini's are long and cylindrical in shape. They are green in color and considered part of the squash family.
Low in carbohydrates, zucchini contains high amounts of vitamin C, potassium and carotenoids (lutein and zeaxanthin).

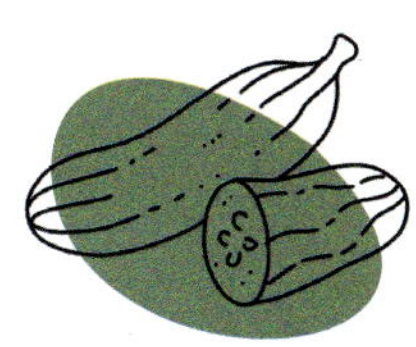

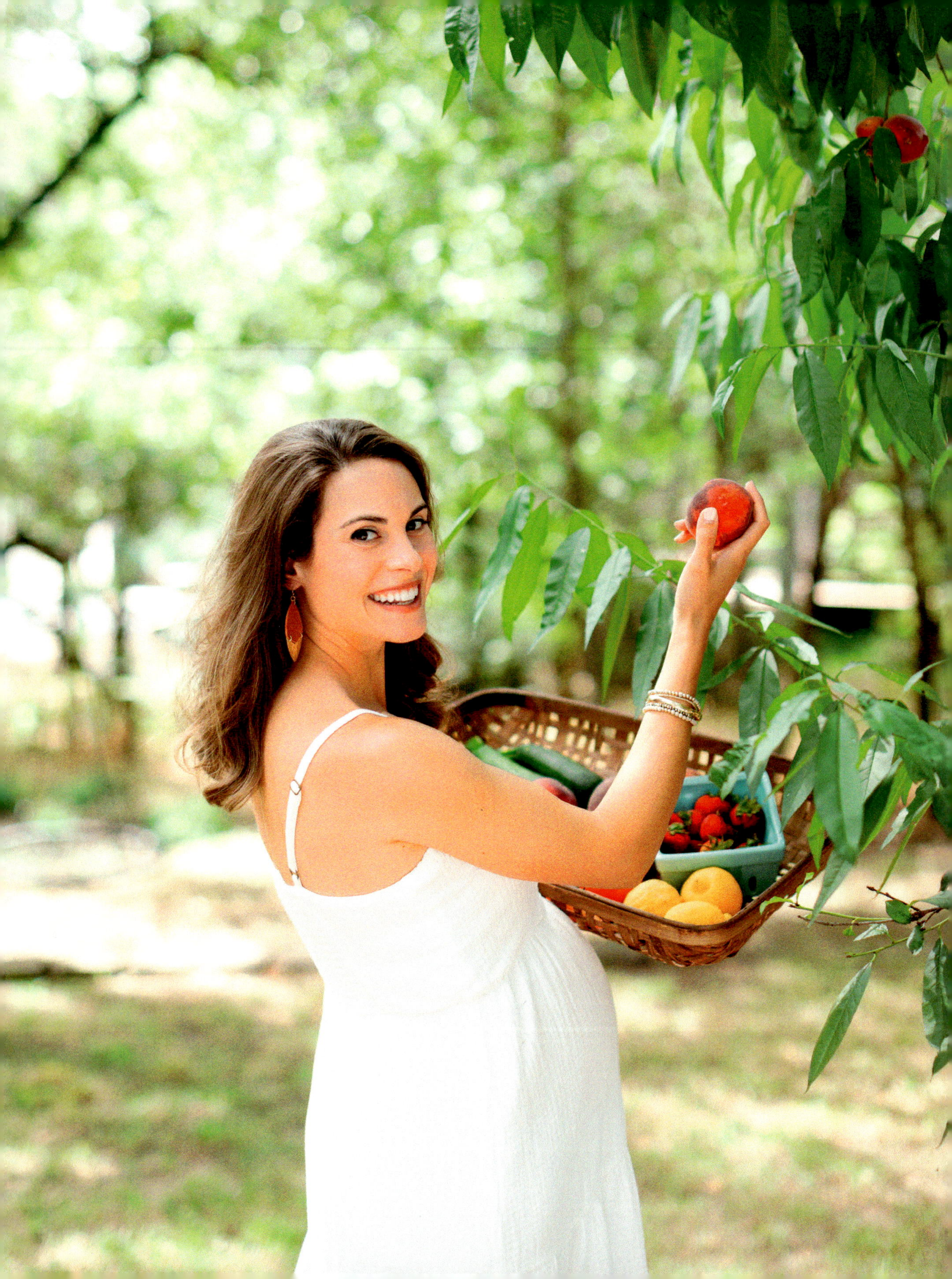

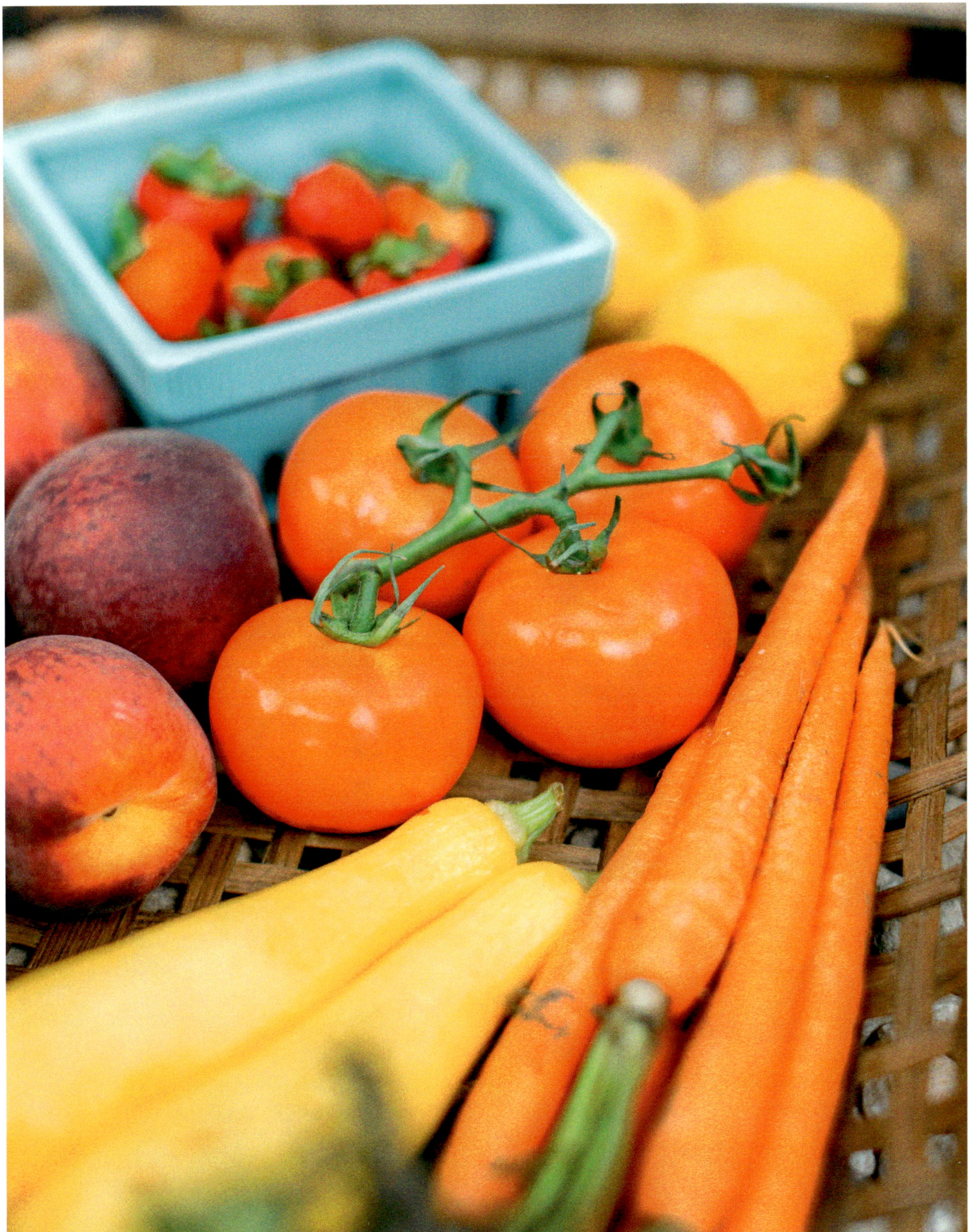

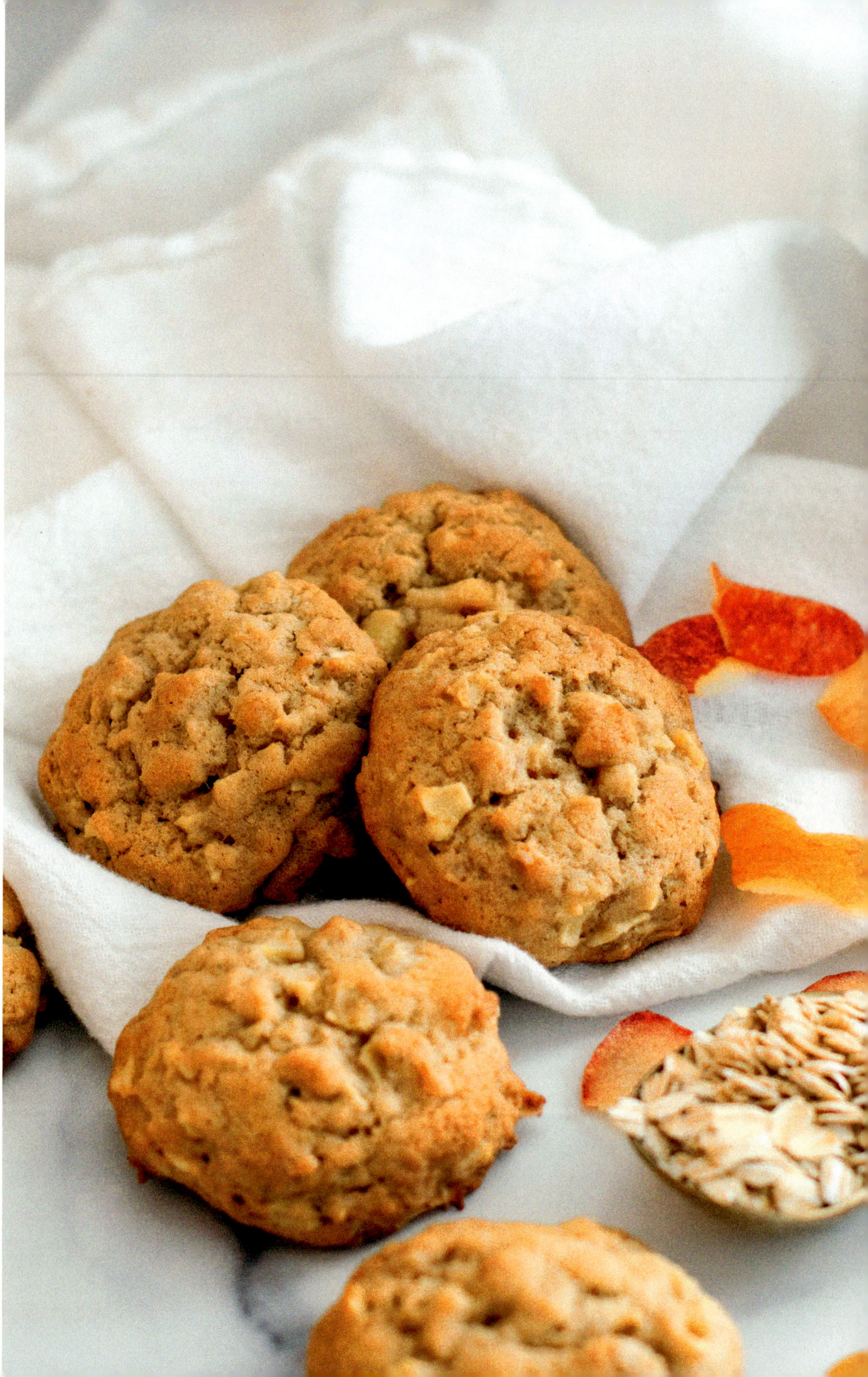

Nut Free

Soy Free

Twice Baked Apple Fritters

One bite and you will be hooked! Whether you like apples or not, it's hard to resist such a fresh tasting cookie. Emmie's favorite part of making these cookies is the apple baking. I chop twice as much as my recipe calls for because she loves dried apples as a snack throughout the week. Best of all they have no added sugar! If you're a mom who likes to multitask like me, this recipe can be made in several simple steps without any stress. Simply chop the apples and get them baking first. Once they have come out of the oven and are cooling, go about the rest of your day until you can come back to them. I've even pre-baked the apples the night before to make the cookies the next day.

PREP TIME: 40 minutes

INACTIVE PREP TIME (apple cooling & dough chilling): 1 hour

COOK TIME: 15 minutes

YIELDS: 18 cookies

Ingredients:

½ cup butter, softened

¼ cup granulated sugar

¼ cup packed light brown sugar

1 large egg

½ tsp vanilla extract

1 ¼ cup all purpose flour

1 tsp pumpkin pie spice

¾ tsp baking soda

Pinch of salt

½ cup old fashioned rolled oats

2 medium sized apples (such as Gala)

Directions:

- Preheat the oven to 350 degrees Fahrenheit and prepare a small baking sheet with parchment paper.
- Skin the apples with a potato skinner and dice into small pieces. Spread out evenly on the prepared baking sheet and bake for 25 minutes. Allow to completely cool (about 1 hour).
- After the apples have cooled, cream together the butter and sugars until light and fluffy (1-2 minutes).
- Add the egg and vanilla extract and continue to mix until combined.
- In a separate mixing bowl mix together the flour, pumpkin pie spice, baking soda, and salt.
- Slowly add the flour mixture to the wet mixture and continue to mix until well-combined.
- Fold in the rolled oats and 1 cup of the cooled baked apples.
- Once dough is combined, place in the fridge to chill for about 15-20 minutes. While dough is chilling, pre-heat the oven to 350 degrees fahrenheit and prepare a baking sheet with parchment paper.
- After the dough has chilled, use a 1 ½ inch cookie scoop to scoop out individual cookies. Place on the cooking sheet.
- Bake for 14-15 minutes or until golden brown

Tips:

Best served warm.

Store in an airtight container for up to 5 days.

☆☆☆☆☆

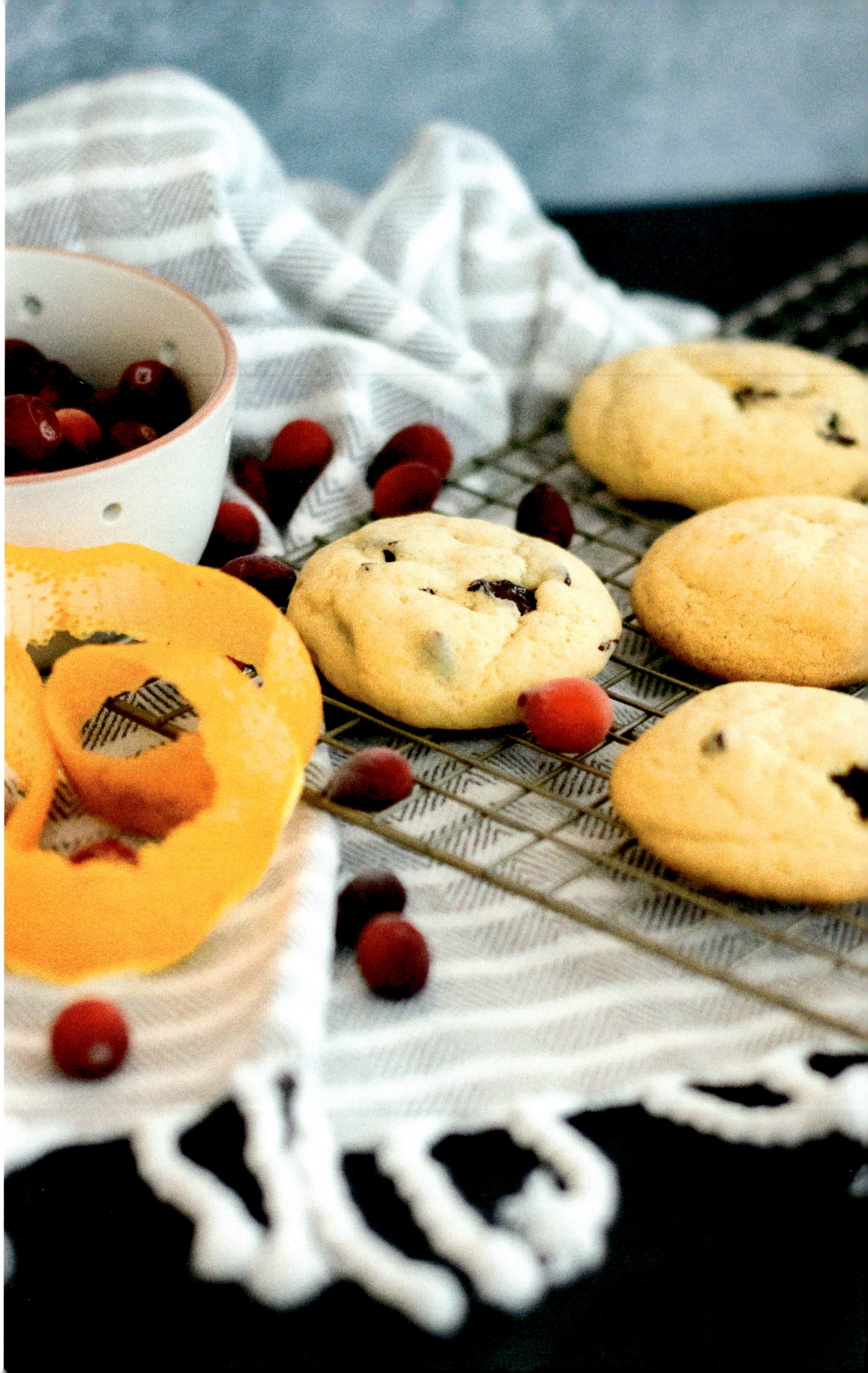

Nut Free

Soy Free

Fresh Squeezed Orange & Cranberry Cookies

Before creating and baking these cookies, my little one had never tasted juice before. We held off giving her juice because most of the juices you find in the grocery stores are saturated with additional sugars that leave you craving more. Until now. While making these cookies, I was fresh squeezing our oranges and Emmie was curious as to what I was doing. I gave her a taste of the fresh squeezed goodness and her eyes lit up like a firecracker was going off in her mouth. In addition to the sweet and indulgent taste, fresh-squeezed orange juice is generous in vitamin C and potassium. I think the best part of making these cookies is not necessarily for the health benefits but letting your little one try fresh-squeezed orange juice for the first time.

OVERALL PREP TIME: 15 minutes

COOK TIME: 13-15 minutes

YIELDS: 20 cookies

Ingredients:

¾ cup butter, softened

½ cup granulated sugar

½ cup packed light brown sugar

1 large egg

1 tsp vanilla extract

2 tbsp grated orange zest

2 tbsp fresh squeezed orange juice

2 ½ cup all purpose flour

½ tsp baking soda

½ tsp baking powder

Pinch of salt

¾ cup dried cranberries

Directions:

PREP: Grate and juice 2 large navel oranges

- Preheat the oven to 350 degrees Fahrenheit. Prepare a baking sheet with parchment paper.
- In a large mixing bowl, cream together the butter and sugars until light and fluffy (about 1-2 minutes). Add the egg and vanilla extract and continue to beat until just combined. Fold in the orange zest and orange juice.
- In a separate mixing bowl, combine the flour, baking soda, baking powder, and pinch of salt.
- Combine the flour mixture with the wet ingredients and mix until well combined.
- Fold in the cranberries
- Roll into 1 inch balls and place on a baking sheet with enough room to spread.
- Bake for 13-15 minutes or until slightly golden brown on the edges and gentle visible cracks appear in the center.

Tip:

Store in an airtight container for up to 1 week.

☆☆☆☆☆

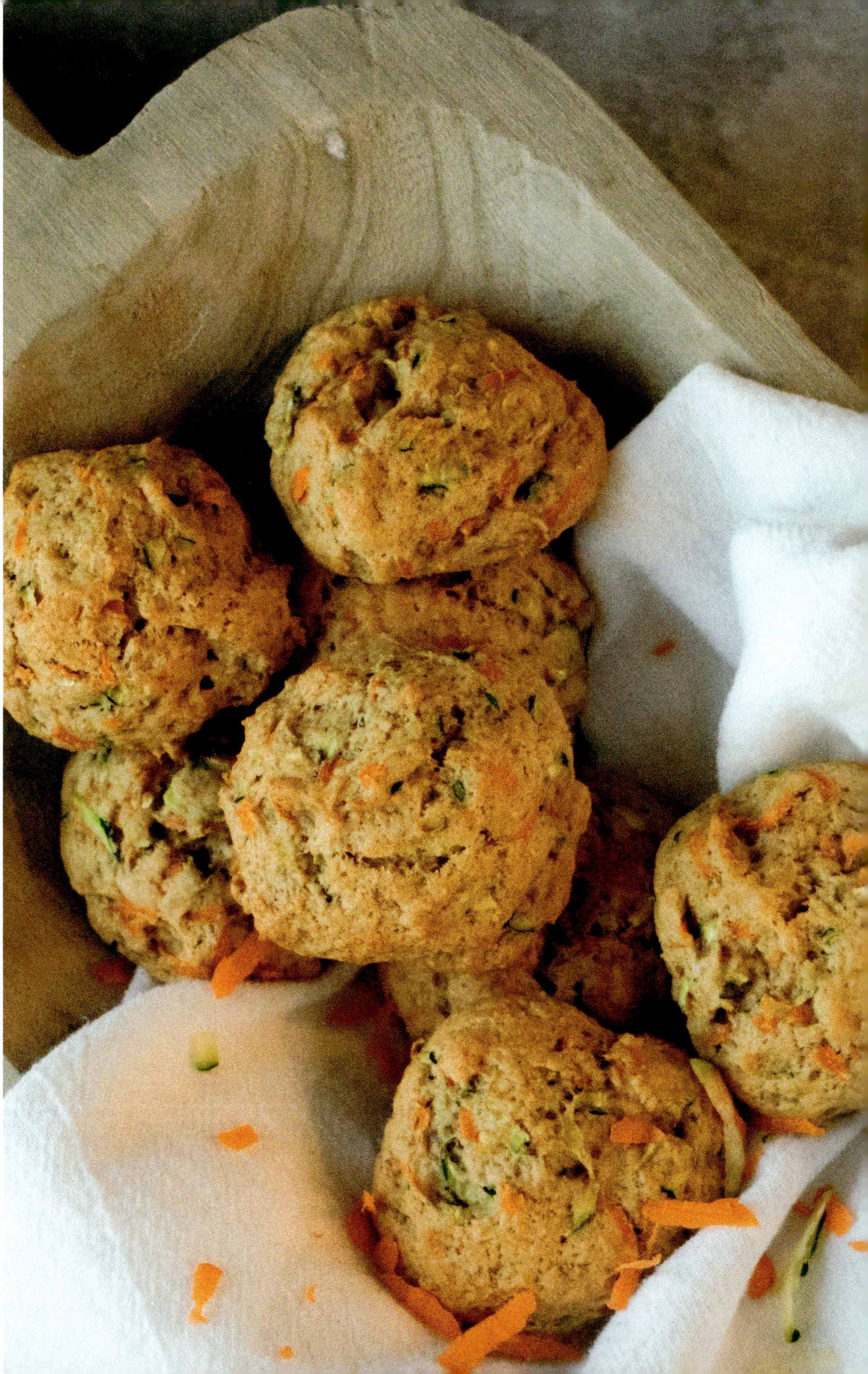

Egg Free

Nut Free

Soy Free

Carrot Zucchini Muffin Cookies

Calling all parents! I've got the perfect cookie for your little one to enjoy while you sit back and smile with pride. Carrots and zucchini are a mighty combo in my house, not only because they go so well together in taste, but they parallel in vitamin profile as well. Carrots and zucchini are both rich in carotenoids, specifically beta-carotene, lutein, and zeaxanthin. These amazing nutrients help promote eye health, among many other benefits. Carrots and zucchini are also rich in vitamin A, vitamin C, fiber, and potassium. Cooking carrots (even in a cookie) helps to break down the cell walls to become bioavailable. That's a great benefit of munching into a delicious cookie bite.

OVERALL PREP TIME: 20 minutes

COOK TIME: 20 minutes

YIELDS: 12-14 cookies

Ingredients:

⅓ cup butter, softened

½ cup packed light brown sugar

1 medium sized banana

1 tsp vanilla extract

1 ¾ cup all purpose flour

½ tsp baking soda

½ tsp baking powder

1 tsp ground cinnamon

¼ tsp salt

½ cup grated zucchini (about 1 medium-sized zucchini)

½ cup grated carrots (about 1 medium-sized carrot)

Directions:

PREP: Mash the banana in a small bowl.

Grate the zucchini using a cheese grater. Using a few paper towels, wrap the grated zucchini to wring out the excess liquid as much as possible. Using the same technique as the zucchini, grate the carrots and wring out the liquid.

- Preheat the oven to 350 degrees Fahrenheit. Prepare a baking sheet with parchment paper.
- In a large mixing bowl, cream together the butter and sugar until light and fluffy (1-2 minutes). Next, add the mashed banana and the vanilla extract. Continue to cream/mix together until well combined.
- In a separate bowl, mix together the flour, baking soda, baking powder, cinnamon, and salt.
- Slowly add the dry flour mixture to the wet ingredients and mix until combined. Next, fold in the zucchini and carrots.
- Roll the dough into 1 ½ inch balls. Place them on a baking sheet and bake for 18 - 20 minutes or until golden brown.

Tips:

Best served warm, same day as baked.

Store in an airtight container for up to 3 days or freeze for up to 3 months

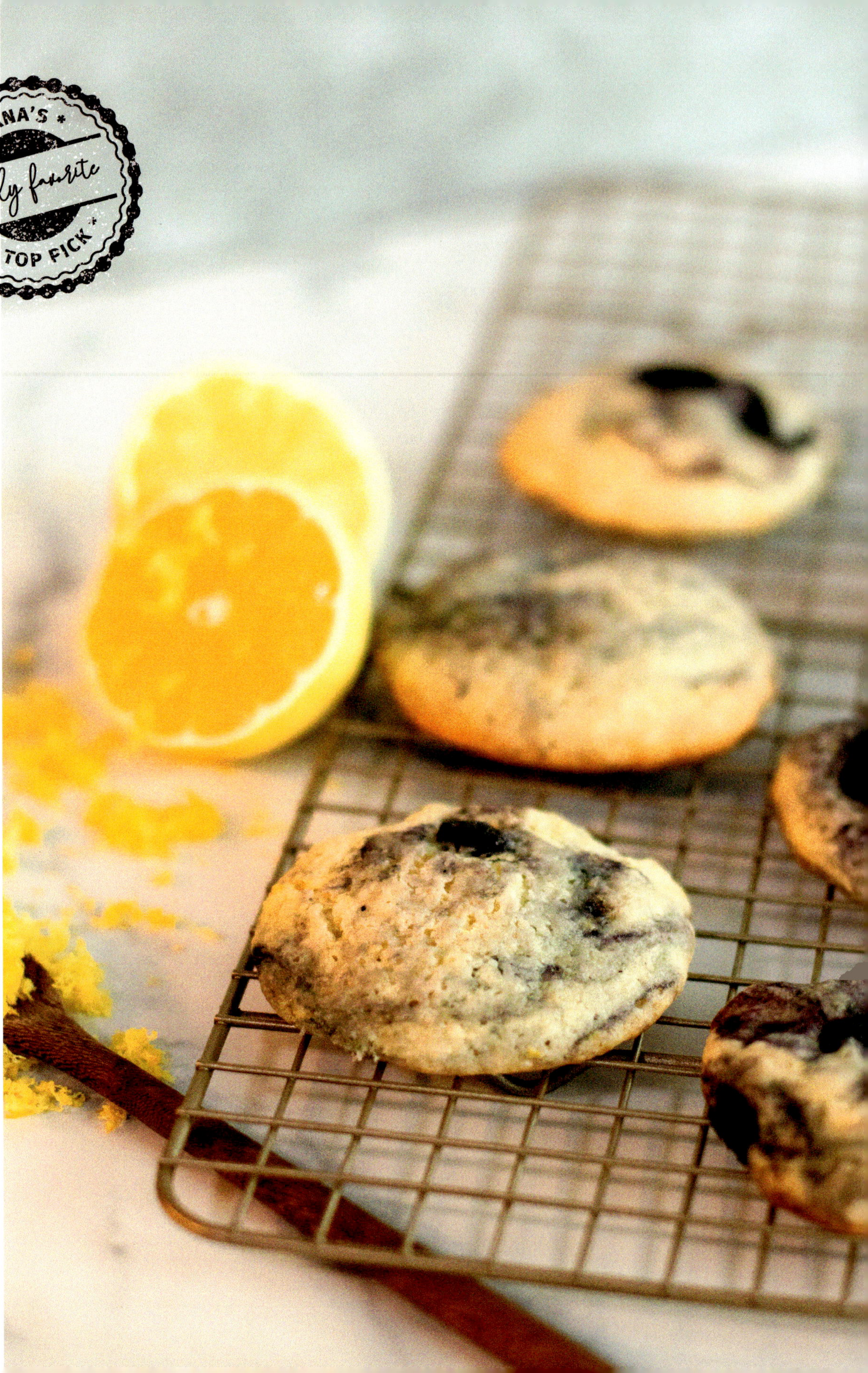

Nut Free

Soy Free

Blueberry Sour Cream Cookies

When I first heard about traditional sour cream cookies, my nose shriveled up in questionable doubt. My guess is that if you've never tried a sour cream cookie, your nose is doing something along the same lines right about now. Nevertheless, I was intrigued when somebody mentioned I ought to make sour cream cookies for this very book. After a few tries in the kitchen, and several taste testings later, I am now a firm believer in putting sour cream in my cookies. The moist and tender texture it creates is unparalleled. If you're looking for a fresh-tasting, ultra moist and tender cookie, this is your golden egg.

Blueberries are rich in antioxidants and provide other health nutrients such as fiber, manganese, vitamin C, and Vitamin K. Together these may help to maintain memory and cognitive function.

OVERALL PREP TIME: 15 - 20 minutes

COOK TIME: 15-16 minutes

YIELDS: 25 cookies

Ingredients:

½ cup butter, softened

1 cup granulated sugar

1 large egg

½ cup sour cream

1 tbsp fresh lemon zest

2 tbsp fresh lemon juice

2 cups all purpose flour

½ cup confectionar's sugar

½ tsp baking soda

½ tsp baking powder

Pinch of salt

1 cup frozen blueberries

Directions:

PREP: Zest and juice 2 large lemons.

- Preheat the oven to 350 degrees Fahrenheit. Prepare a baking sheet with parchment paper.
- In a large mixing bowl, cream together the butter and sugar until light and fluffy (about 1-2 minutes). Add the egg and continue to beat. Add the sour cream and continue to beat. Do not overmix.
- Fold in the lemon zest and lemon juice.
- In a separate mixing bowl, combine the flour, confectionar's sugar, baking soda, baking powder, and pinch of salt.
- Combine the flour mixture to the wet ingredients and mix until well combined.
- Fold in the blueberries until just combined. Do not overmix.
- Using a Scoop #100, scoop out balls of dough onto the prepared baking sheet with enough room to slightly spread. The dough will be loose, like muffin batter.
- Bake for 15-16 minutes or until the bottoms get very lightly browned and visible cracking is seen in the middle of the cookie.

Tip:

Store in an airtight container for up to 7 days.

☆☆☆☆☆

TATA'S
family favorite
TOP PICK

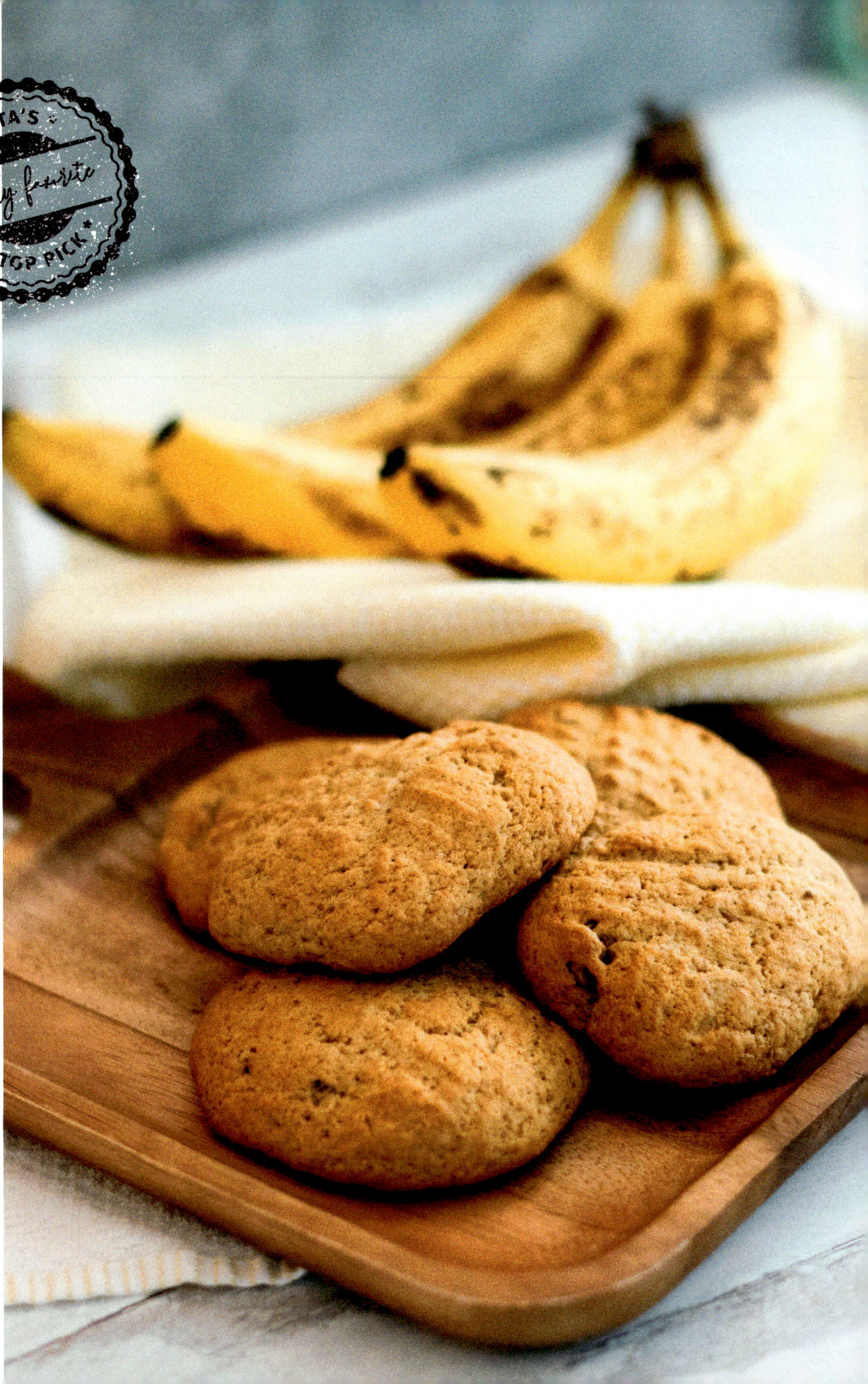

Egg Free

Soy Free

Banana Bread Walnut Cookies

Who doesn't love the smell and taste of fresh baked banana bread? The day my countertop bananas turn slightly browned and mushy is one of the best days at my house. On this day, our trusty midafternoon snack smeared with almond butter will turn into something a bit more glamorous with the help of a few extra ingredients (flour, butter, cinnamon, & vanilla). However, before racing to put these cookies in the oven, don't forget those healthy walnuts as well. Walnuts are packed with iron, magnesium, vitamin E, phosphorus, and antioxidants. Although I think walnuts' most notable health benefits are the polyunsaturated fats, which are rich in omega-3 fatty acids such as alpha linolenic acid. Together, these may benefit heart health by reducing LDL cholesterol, diabetes, metabolic syndrome, aging effects, and increasing cognitive health.

OVERALL PREP TIME: 15 minutes

INACTIVE PREP TIME: 20 mins to chill dough

COOK TIME: 13-15 minutes

YIELDS: 15 cookies

Ingredients:

½ cup butter, softened

½ cup granulated sugar

½ cup mashed banana (about 1 ½ medium bananas)

1 tsp vanilla extract

1 ¾ cup all purpose flour

½ tsp baking soda

½ tsp baking powder

1 tsp ground cinnamon

Pinch of salt

⅓ cup finely chopped walnuts

Directions:

PREP: Mash the bananas in a small bowl.

- Preheat the oven to 375 degrees Fahrenheit. Prepare a baking sheet with parchment paper.
- In a large mixing bowl, cream together the butter and sugar until light and fluffy (about 1-2 minutes). Add the mashed banana and vanilla extract.
- In a separate mixing bowl, combine the flour, baking soda, baking powder, ground cinnamon, and pinch of salt.
- Combine the flour mixture to the wet ingredients and mix until well combined.
- Fold in the walnuts
- Place the dough in the fridge to chill for about 20-25 minutes.
- Roll into 1 inch balls and place on a baking sheet. Using a fork, lightly smash the dough ball down in 2 different directions (like you would with a peanut butter cookie).
- Bake for 13-15 minutes or until golden brown.

Tips:

Best served warm the day they are baked.

Store in an airtight container for up to 3 days.

☆☆☆☆☆

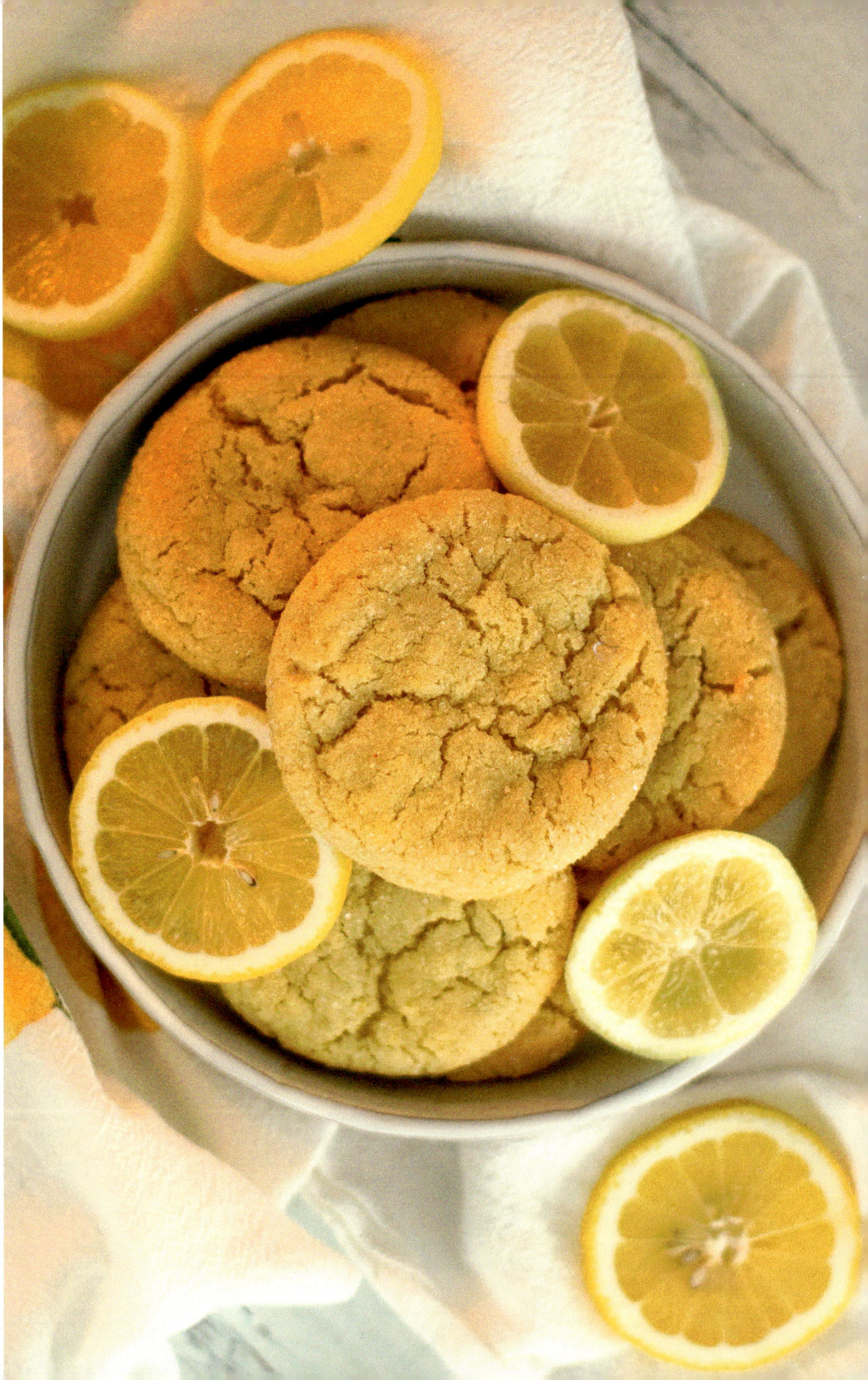

Nut Free

Soy Free

Pucker Up Lemon Sugar Cookies

Sunday evenings are spent at my in-laws house. It's been a tradition of ours since before Emmie was born and we keep it up even when life tries to get in the way. My mother-in-law, Mimi, does the cooking and I bring the dessert. I've always said it's the perfect way to unwind from the past week, catching up on what happened, and recharging for the upcoming week. It's a special time for Emmie to run loose in their backyard, and if it's a warm summer evening we usually end up in the pool by the end of the evening. We joked a while back that I should name this cookbook, "Sundays at Mimi's", because for as long as we've been going, I've been bringing a sweet dessert to end the night on. These lemon cookies are among our favorites, they are fresh-tasting and so easy to whip up the day you need them: perfect for a Sunday spent with family and friends.

OVERALL PREP TIME: 20 minutes

COOK TIME: 12-13 minutes

YIELDS: 24 cookies

Ingredients:

1 cup butter, softened

1 ½ cup granulated sugar

3 heaping tbsp fresh lemon zest (about 3 large lemons)

3 tbsp fresh lemon juice

1 large egg

3 cups all purpse flour

2 tsp baking soda

Pinch of salt

1 cup granulated sugar to roll the cookies in before baking

Directions:

PREP: Zest and juice 3 large lemons.

- Preheat the oven to 350 degrees Fahrenheit. Prepare 2 baking sheets with parchment paper.
- In a large mixing bowl, cream together the butter and sugar until light and fluffy (about 1-2 minutes). Add the lemon zest, lemon juice, and egg and continue mixing until incorporated. Do not overmix.
- In a separate mixing bowl, combine the flour, baking soda, and salt.
- Pouring half at a time, combine the flour mixture to the wet ingredients and mix until well combined.
- Pour the remaining sugar into a small bowl for rolling cookies.
- Roll dough into individual 1½ inch balls, and then roll in the sugar before placing them on the baking sheet. Allow for the dough to spread.
- Bake for 12-13 minutes or until golden brown with slight cracking tops.

Tip:

Store on the counter in an airtight container for up to 6 days.

☆☆☆☆☆

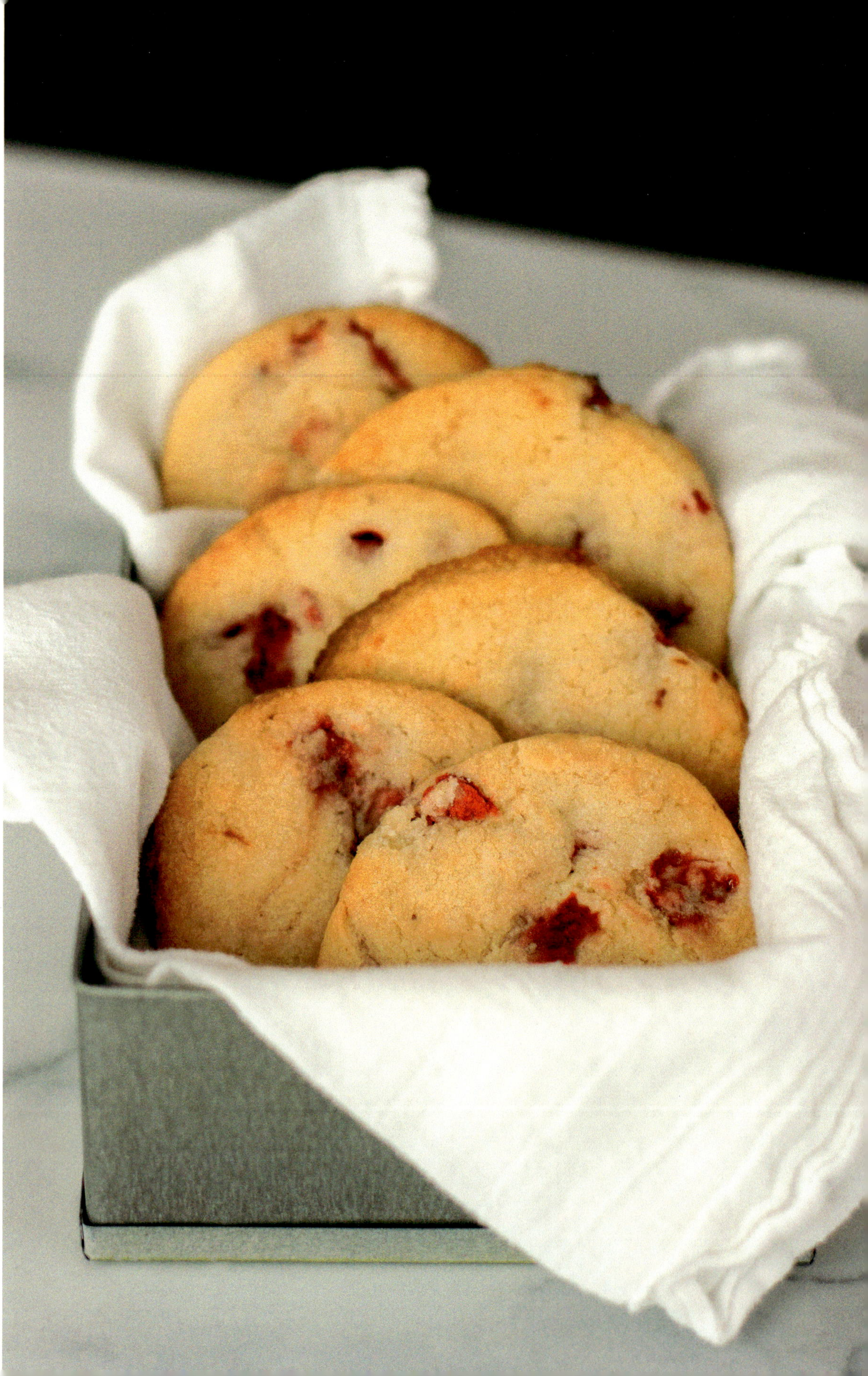

Egg Free

Nut Free

Soy Free

Summertime Strawberry Scone Cookies

There's nothing that excites me more than when the sweet Texas strawberry season has finally arrived. I've gone to pick fresh strawberries from local patches for a few years now and it's become one of my favorite things to look forward to all year long. There's nothing quite like a fresh-picked strawberry, it's incomparable to that of a store-bought strawberry. Not only are strawberries mouthwatering, but the health benefits are multitudinous. They are a great source of vitamin C, fiber, and folate, all of which are essential to our health and wellbeing (especially if you're pregnant). A diet rich in strawberries can also help to lower total and LDL cholesterol and lower your risk of stroke and cardiovascular disease. The bright red pigment comes from a phytonutrient called anthocyanin, which provides the antioxidant and anti-inflammatory health benefits. When I don't go to the local patches, I try to find strawberries in the store with deep red coloring from tip to stem. So go ahead, search out the best strawberries and get to baking up something sweet without much guilt. I hope you enjoy these summertime strawberry scone cookies as much as my mother-in-law and I do.

OVERALL PREP TIME: 25 minutes

COOK TIME: 18-20 minutes

YIELDS: 16 cookies

Ingredients:

2 ¾ cup all purpose flour

1 tsp baking powder

1 cup packed confectioner's sugar

½ cup granulated sugar

Pinch of salt

½ cup heavy whipping cream

1 tsp pure vanilla extract

1 cup cold butter, cut into tbsp pieces

1 cup diced strawberries, chilled

Tip:

Store in an airtight container either in the fridge or countertop for up to 5 days.

Directions:

- Preheat the oven to 375 degrees Fahrenheit. Prepare 2 baking sheets with parchment paper.
- In an extra-large mixing bowl, whisk together the flour, baking powder, confectioner's sugar, granulated sugar, and salt. Set aside.
- In a separate small mixing bowl, whisk together the heavy cream and vanilla extract. Set aside.
- Using a pastry cutter, cut the cold butter into the flour mixture until the flour resembles tiny peas and is consistent throughout.
- Pour in the heavy cream mixture, using a sturdy spatula. Begin incorporating the dough together as much as possible. Once the dough gets thick and unable to easily use the spatula, begin using your hands to knead the dough. The dough starts out very tough to combine and you will be tempted to add more liquid. But don't! It's important to keep kneading the dough as is. Keep shaping until all the flour has been incorporated (may take about 5-8 minutes of manually kneading). It should come together to form one large heavy dough ball, if there is dry flour still in the mixing bowl, keep working it. This takes some muscle, but you've got this!
- Lastly, fold in the chilled strawberries. The dough will become slightly sticky/ slippery due to the extra moisture. Do not overwork the dough at this point.
- Roll the dough out on a generously floured surface (I prefer to use a slipmat for easier clean up) until about ½ inch thick. Using a biscuit cutter (your choice of size; I used a 3" diameter cutter), cut out the cookies and place on the prepared baking sheets. You will have excess dough after cutting, simply remold and reroll the dough for more cookies.
- Bake for 18-20 minutes or until golden brown and desired texture is achieved. *I prefer to have slightly more crunchy scones (20 minutes) but softer scones are excellent as well (18 minutes).*

☆☆☆☆☆

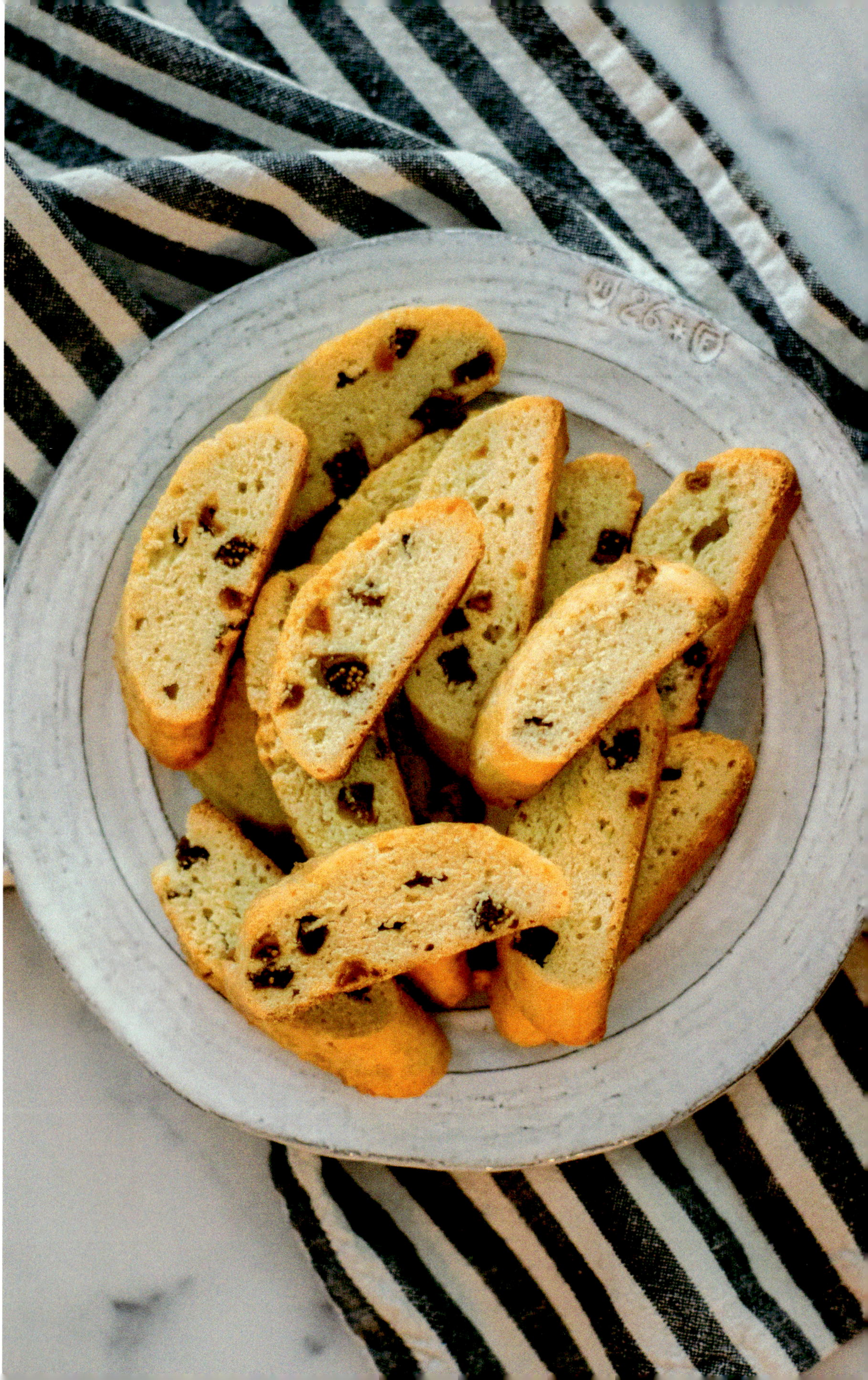

Nut Free

Soy Free

Get Figgy With It - Breakfast Biscotti

Cookies for breakfast? Yes, I dare say, you can have a cookie (or two) for breakfast and still live a balanced and healthy life. These fig biscotti cookies are perfect for munching on paired with your strong morning brew or freshly steeped tea. I wanted to incorporate dried figs in this biscotti because the taste and nutrient profile just seemed fitting. Dried figs are exceptionally sweet yet earthy, making the biscotti tasteful without overpowering the simplicity and tradition of the recipe. My daughter, Emmie and I love to munch on dried figs as a snack, or as additions to my salad or her lunch plate. The nutrient density of a fig is one to mention as well. These little guys are excellent sources of magnesium, manganese, and soluble fiber. Figs also have an abundance of heart healthy polyphenols making them a powerhouse. Maybe I should have added more figs to the recipe? I'll let you decide. In the meantime, I hope you enjoy these sweet, slightly earthy, biscotti cookies for breakfast without any guilt.

OVERALL PREP TIME: 15 minutes

COOK TIME: 38-40 minutes

YIELDS: 26-27 Biscotti pieces

Ingredients:

½ cup butter, softened

½ cup granulated sugar

2 large eggs

2 tsp pure vanilla extract

2 cups all purpose flour

½ tsp baking powder

Pinch of salt

½ cup dried, finely chopped figs

1 large egg white, beaten

Turbinado sugar for sprinkling on top

Directions:

- Preheat the oven to 350 degrees Fahrenheit. Prepare 1 baking sheet with parchment paper.
- In a small mixing bowl, whisk together the flour, baking powder, and salt. Set aside.
- In a separate mixing bowl using an electric mixer, cream together the butter and sugar until light and fluffy (about 1-3 minutes). Add the eggs, one at a time making sure to beat well on low speed between each. Add the vanilla extract and continue to beat on low.
- Add the dry flour mixture, ½ at a time, to the wet ingredients and continue to mix until the dough is smooth and consistent.
- Fold in the chopped figs.
- Using your hands, divide the dough into 2 equal portions. Place one portion on the prepared baking sheet and gently roll/shape into a cylindrical log about 1 foot long and 1 ½ inches wide. Repeat with the second dough portion, placing on the same baking sheet. Allow room for the dough to rise/spread slightly.
- Brush the dough logs with the beaten egg white and sprinkle turbinado sugar generously all over.
- Bake for 28-30 minutes. After baking, pull the baking sheet out of the oven, without turning the oven off let the dough cool for 10 minutes. After 10 minutes, using a serrated bread knife, slice the dough diagonally into ½ inch slices.
- Spread the slices out on the baking sheet, side down, and continue to bake for another 12-14 minutes.

Tip:

Can be stored in the open air or in an airtight container for up to 7 days.

☆☆☆☆☆

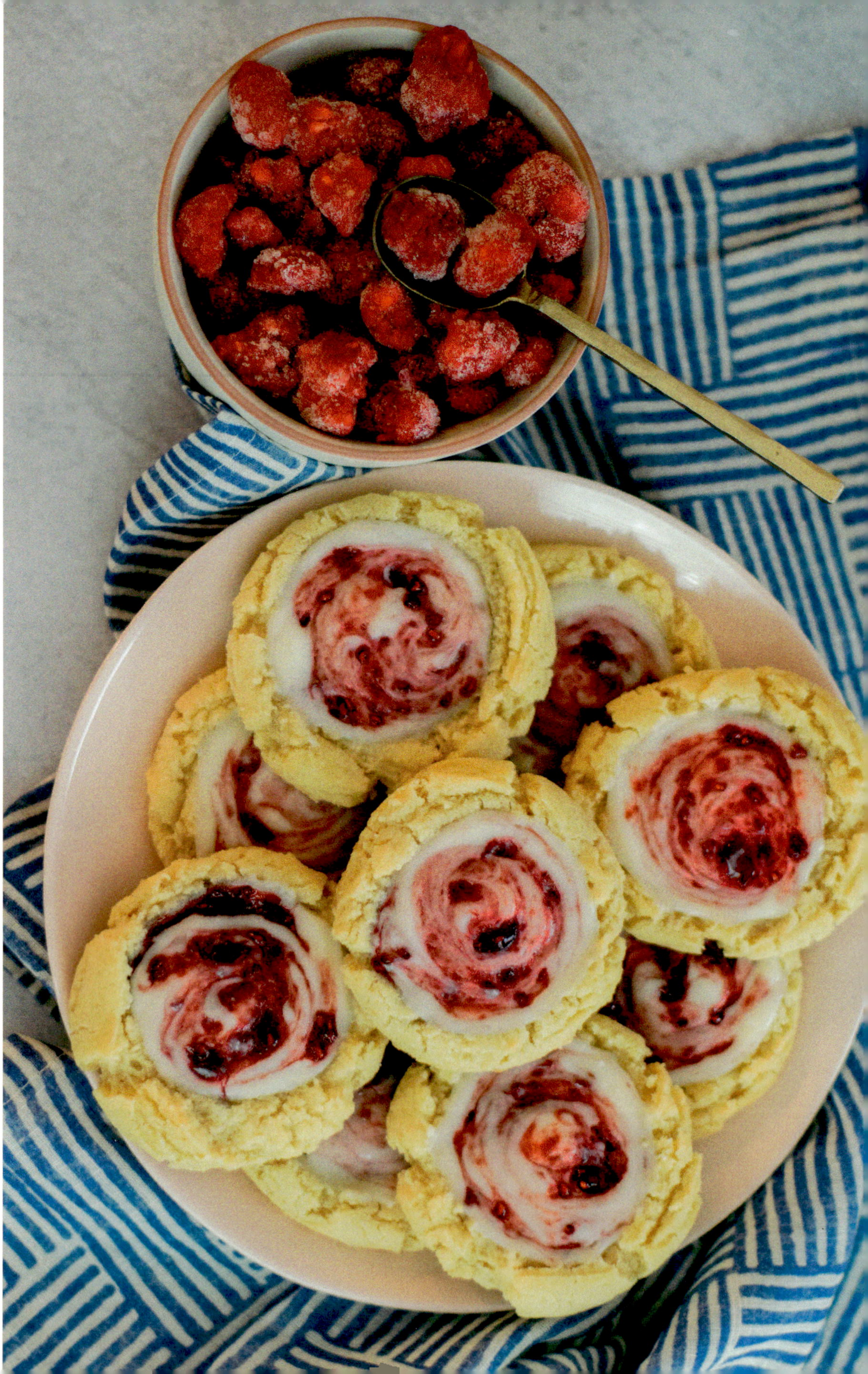

Nut Free

Soy Free

Decadent Raspberry Cream Cheese Danish Cookies

These cookies hold a special place in my heart because I spent an entire week making sure they were perfect enough to include in this book. I think I even had dreams about these cookies at one point. If you don't know, I am a sucker for cream cheese and just about anything that resembles a danish. Together, the soft cookie and cream cheese filling create a beautiful balance that can only be described as rich and decadent. Beyond the obvious delicious taste of these cookies, they are also perfect for entertaining during a party or shower. Try using different fruit preserves such as blueberry, orange and apricot, etc. to create different colors to celebrate. The key to making these cookies the best they can be is to pull them out of the oven BEFORE they turn golden brown like a traditional cookie.

PREP TIME: 25 minutes

CHILL TIME: 1 hour

TOTAL COOK TIME: 17 minutes

YIELDS: 24-26 cookies

Ingredients:

FOR THE COOKIES

1 cup butter, softened

1 ½ cup granulated sugar

1 large egg

1 tsp pure vanilla extract

3 cups all purpose flour

2 tsp baking soda

Pinch of coarse kosher salt

FOR THE FILLING

8 oz soft cream cheese

½ cup confectioner's sugar

½ tsp pure vanilla extract

⅓ cup raspberry preserves

Tips:

Store in the fridge for up to 6-7 days.

Swap out the raspberry preserves for any other fruit preserves to create a different taste, such as strawberry, apricot, blueberry or orange.

Directions:

- In a large mixing bowl using an electric mixer, cream together the butter and sugar until light and fluffy (about 3-4 minutes). Add the egg and vanilla extract and continue mixing until incorporated.
- In a separate mixing bowl, combine the flour, baking soda, and salt.
- Pouring half at a time, combine the flour mixture to the wet ingredients and mix until well combined. You may need to use a spatula to finish incorporating the dough by hand.
- Roll dough into individual 1 ½ inch balls, placing them on a baking sheet. You will chill the dough before cooking so there is no need for spacing them out yet.
- Cover with plastic wrap and place the baking sheet in the refrigerator to chill for 1 hour.
- While the cookies are chilling, prep the cream cheese filling. Using the electric mixer, cream together the softened cream cheese, confectioner's sugar, and vanilla until smooth and creamy. Set aside for later.
- Once the cookies are done chilling, preheat the oven to 350 degrees Fahrenheit. Prepare 2 baking sheets with parchment paper.
- Place pre-portioned chilled cookies on the prepared baking sheet (Cookies will spread slightly but not much so space accordingly).
- Bake for 10 minutes. Pull the cookies out of the oven. Using the bottom of a small flat glass or ¼ cup measuring cup, press into the soft/warm cookie to create a bowl-like shape.
- Scoop 1 large tsp of the cream cheese filling and ½ tsp raspberry preserves into each bowl created. Using a toothpick, swirl the raspberry preserves into the cream cheese, creating an artistic effect. Repeat with the remaining cookies on the sheet.
- Place cookies back in the oven to continue baking for another 7 minutes. Do not overcook.

☆☆☆☆☆

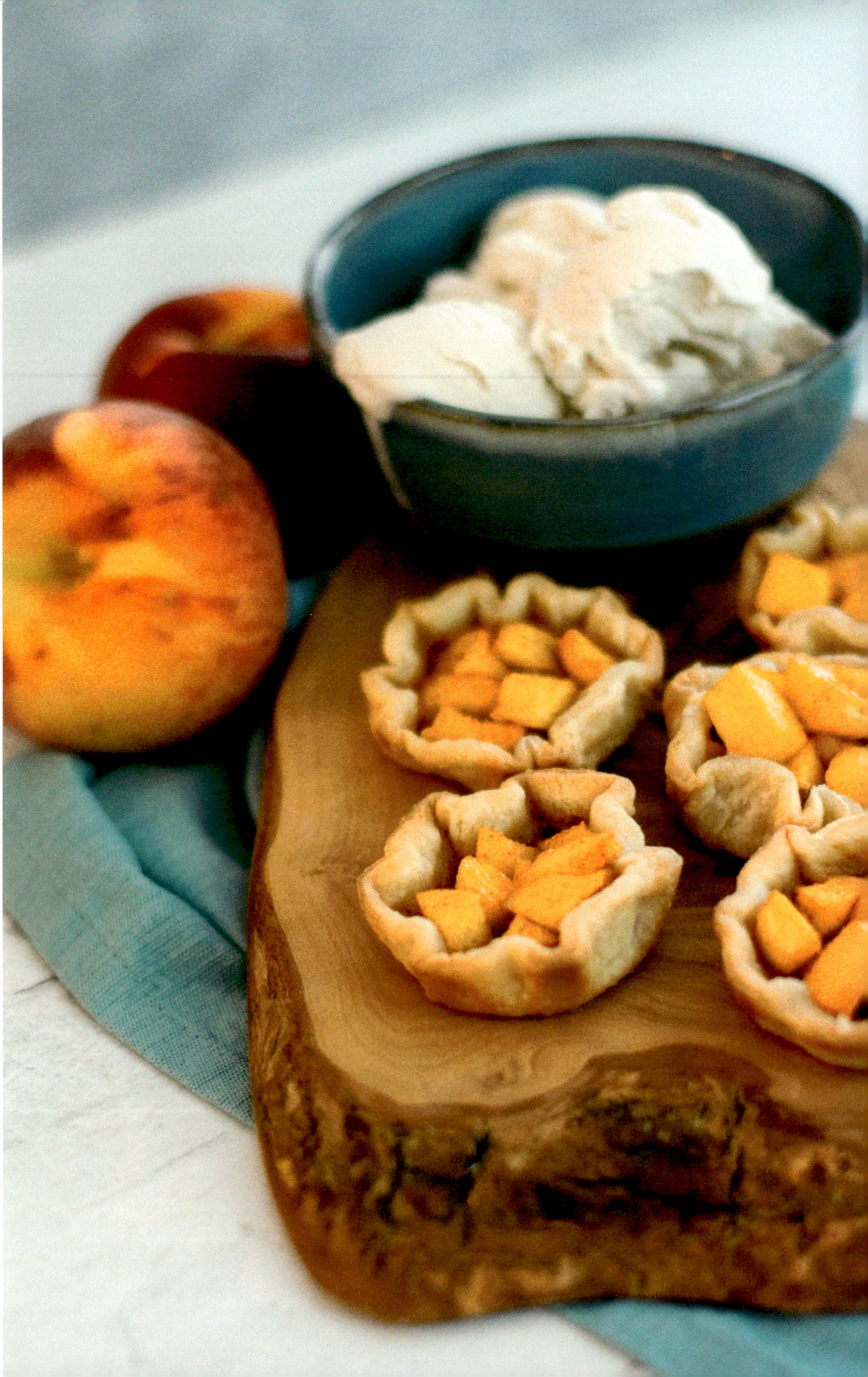

Nut Free

Soy Free

Mini Peach Pie Cookie Cups

Fresh peaches in the summertime remind me of simple times. Simple times as a kid when one bite of a fresh peach would send the juice running all the way down your chin and into your hands. Although I've always lived in Texas and the hill country can produce some amazing fresh peaches, I can only imagine what the peaches from the true South taste like. I imagine they taste like candy, exploding with flavor and juices that make you salivate for them every summer to come. The options to incorporate peaches in dessert are endless: peach cobbler, peach flambé, peach pie, peach ice cream, peaches n' cream, grilled peaches you name it! To me there's nothing more southern than a backyard BBQ finished with a slice of warm peach cobbler and homemade vanilla ice cream. These bite-sized peach pie cookie cups aim to mimic that tradition, plus the individual portions make them great for parties or family get-togethers. Serve them warm with a dollop of vanilla ice cream or whipped cream and you've got yourself a dessert that will leave your guests asking for more.

TOTAL PREP TIME: 50 minutes (includes soak time)

INACTIVE PREP TIME/SOAK TIME: 30 minutes

COOK TIME: 20-22 minutes

YIELDS: 18 mini-pie cookies

Ingredients:

2 sheets store-bought prepared pie dough, rolled out

1 ½ cup fresh peaches, skinned and cut into small cubes

½ cup granulated sugar

1 tsp ground cinnamon

Optional:
Vanilla ice cream or whipped cream

Directions:

- Preheat the oven to 350 degrees Fahrenheit and lightly grease the bottom of 2 muffin tins.
- In a small mixing bowl, combine the cubed peaches, granulated sugar, and ground cinnamon. Mix together and let sit for 30 mins. After 30 minutes, drain the excess liquid but do not discard.
- Using a large biscuit cutter (about 3" diameter) or a large-mouth drinking glass, cut circles in the rolled out pie dough.
- Spoon out a small serving (6-8 pieces) of the peach cube mixture to place in the center of each dough circle. Using your fingers, pinch the dough together to form a tight edge all the way around. This prevents the peach cubes from spilling out.
- Transfer the pinched mini pies to the prepared muffin tins. Using a spoon, pour a small amount of reserved peach liquid into each mini pie. Don't overfill with liquid or it will cause the bottom to burn.
- Bake 20-22 minutes or until the pie dough becomes slightly golden brown and the dough is slightly firm to the touch.
- Serve warm with a scoop of vanilla ice cream or whipped cream.

Tips:

Store in the fridge for up to one week. Simply rewarm when ready to enjoy

Consider adding a dutch crumble topping if you're wanting more cookie sweetness (simply combine brown sugar, cinnamon, butter, and flour together). Crumble on top of the peach cubes before baking.

☆☆☆☆☆

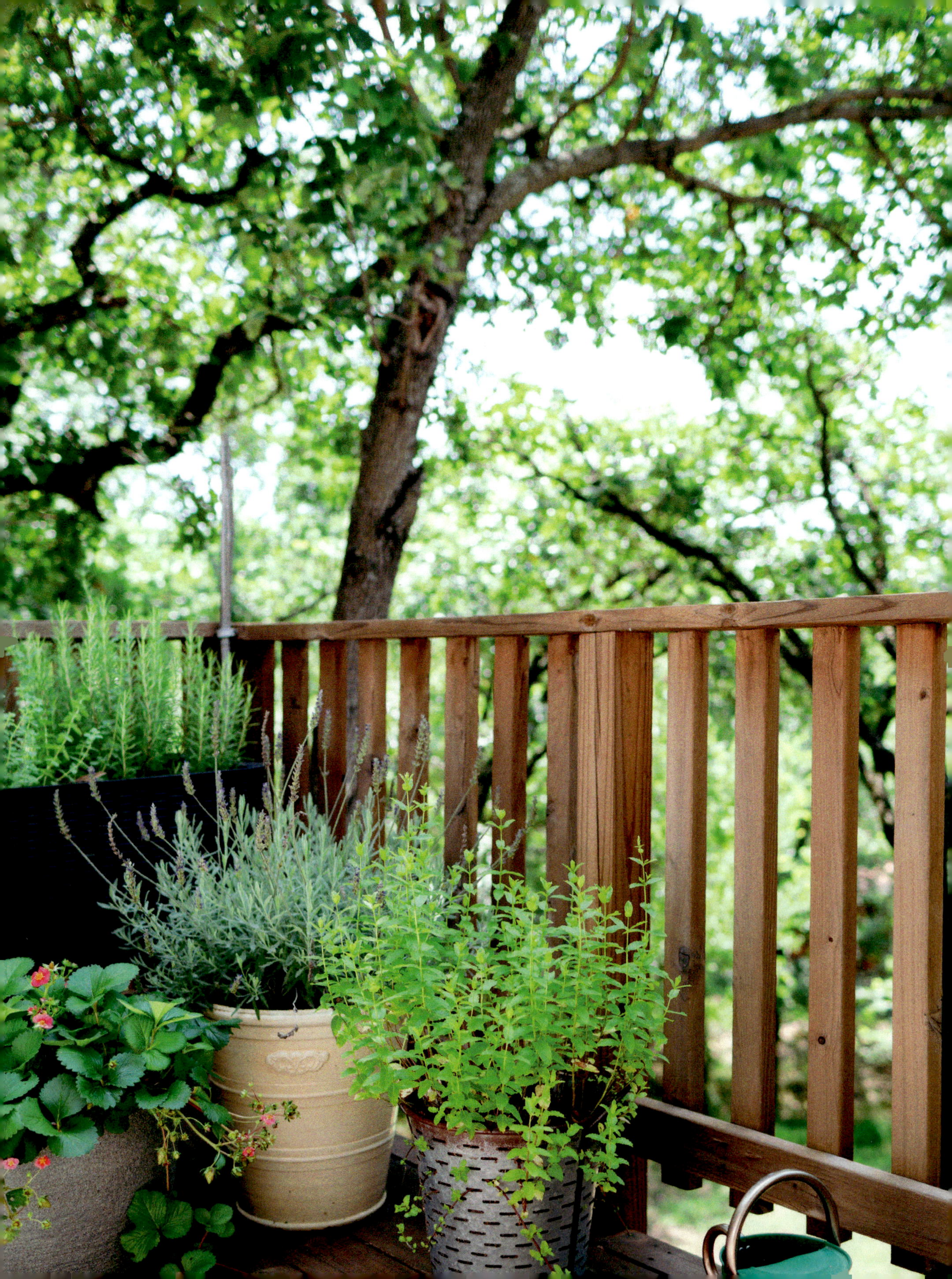

Sweet & Savory herb Garden delights

- Mother Earth Lavender Shortbread Cookies
- Oregano & Rosemary Butter Cookies
- Double Chocolate Garden Mint Cookies *(Nana's Pick)*
- Chai Tea Latte Cookies
- Savory Rosemary Parmesan Shortbread Cookies
- Mini Cheddar and Chive Crackers
- Simply Sweet Chamomile Tea Cookies

Herb Classification

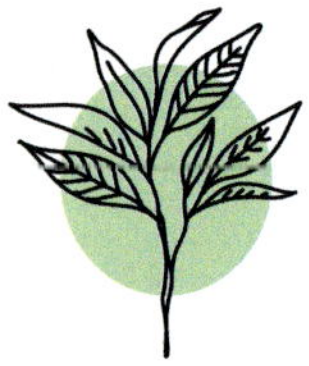

Chai

Camellia sinensis

Chai is a collection of warm spices including cinnamon, ginger, cardamom, black pepper, nutmeg, and cloves. A classic Chai tea tastes both sweet and spicy.

The blend of spices are known for health benefits such as reducing the risk for heart disease, reducing blood sugar levels, and improving overall digestion.

Chamomile

Matricaria chamomilla

Typically grows in nature with an appearance similar to daises. Chamomile is slightly bitter in taste.

Used for indigestion, insomnia, and ailments such as colds & fevers. Can be used externally for burns and rashes.

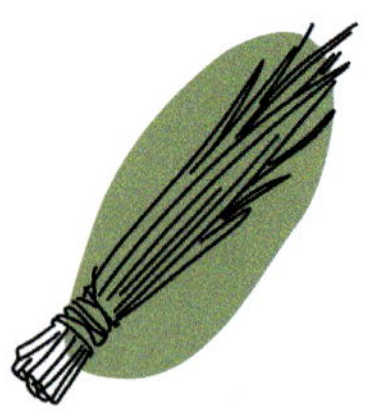

Chives

Allium schoenoprasum

Grows edible long, skinny-stemmed leaves and flowers. This herb has a mild onion flavor that is not to be confused with green onions.

Contains vitamin K, folate, and carotenoids such as lutein and zeaxanthin.

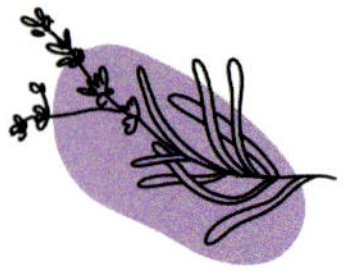

Lavender

Lavandula angustifolia

Grows best in the sunshine and produces purple, long stemmed flowers. Aromatic, pungent & bitter in taste.

Used for bacterial and fungal infections. Can also be used for anxiety, pain, wounds, headaches and relieving depression.

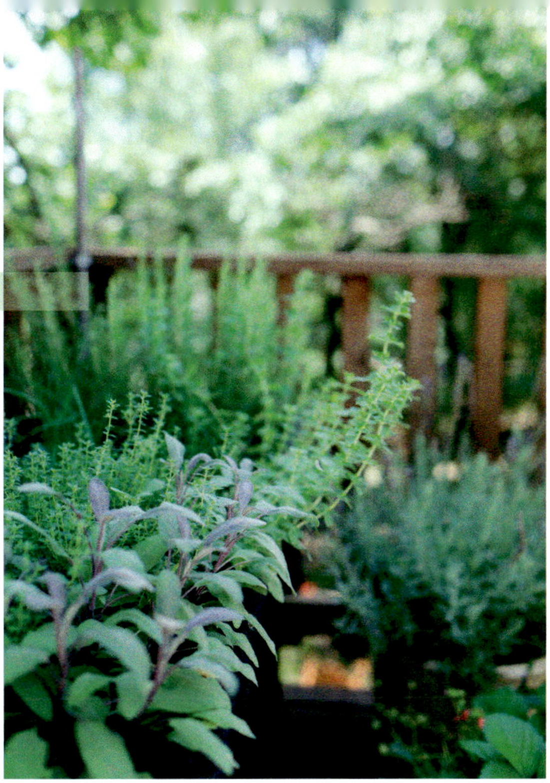

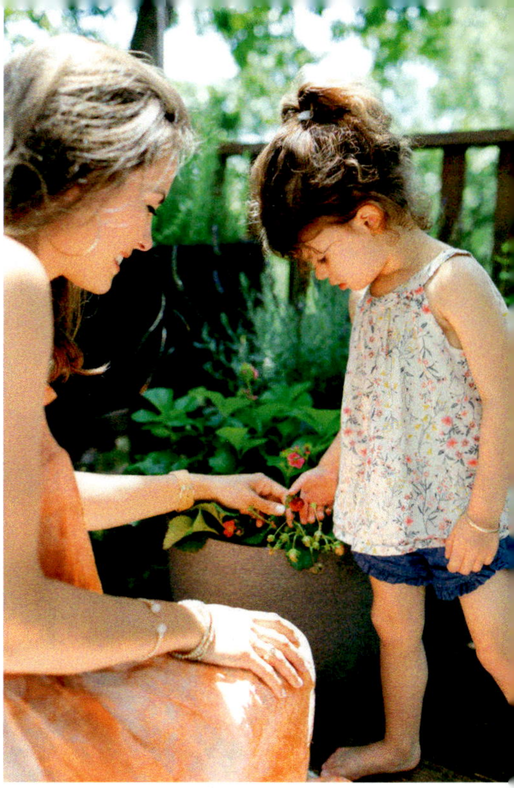

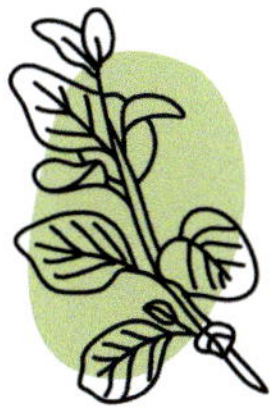

Oregano

Origanum vulgare

Easy to grow flowering herb in the mint family. Oregano has a woody, pungent taste used traditionally in Greek, Roman, and Italian cooking.

Oregano has wonderful health benefits that have been used for centuries both topically and when ingested. Contains antioxidants and antibacterial properties.

Peppermint

Mentha x piperita

Fast growing herb that produces small, bright green leaves. Taste is strong and pungent.

Used for upset stomachs, hiccups, and relieving sinus congestion, gas, nausea, and headaches. Can be used externally to reduce inflammation and itching of the skin.

Rosemary

Rosmarinus officinalis

Easy-to-grow herb with branch-like leaves. Warm and pungent taste profile.

Used for digestion, skin protection, food perseveration, and mental stimulation.

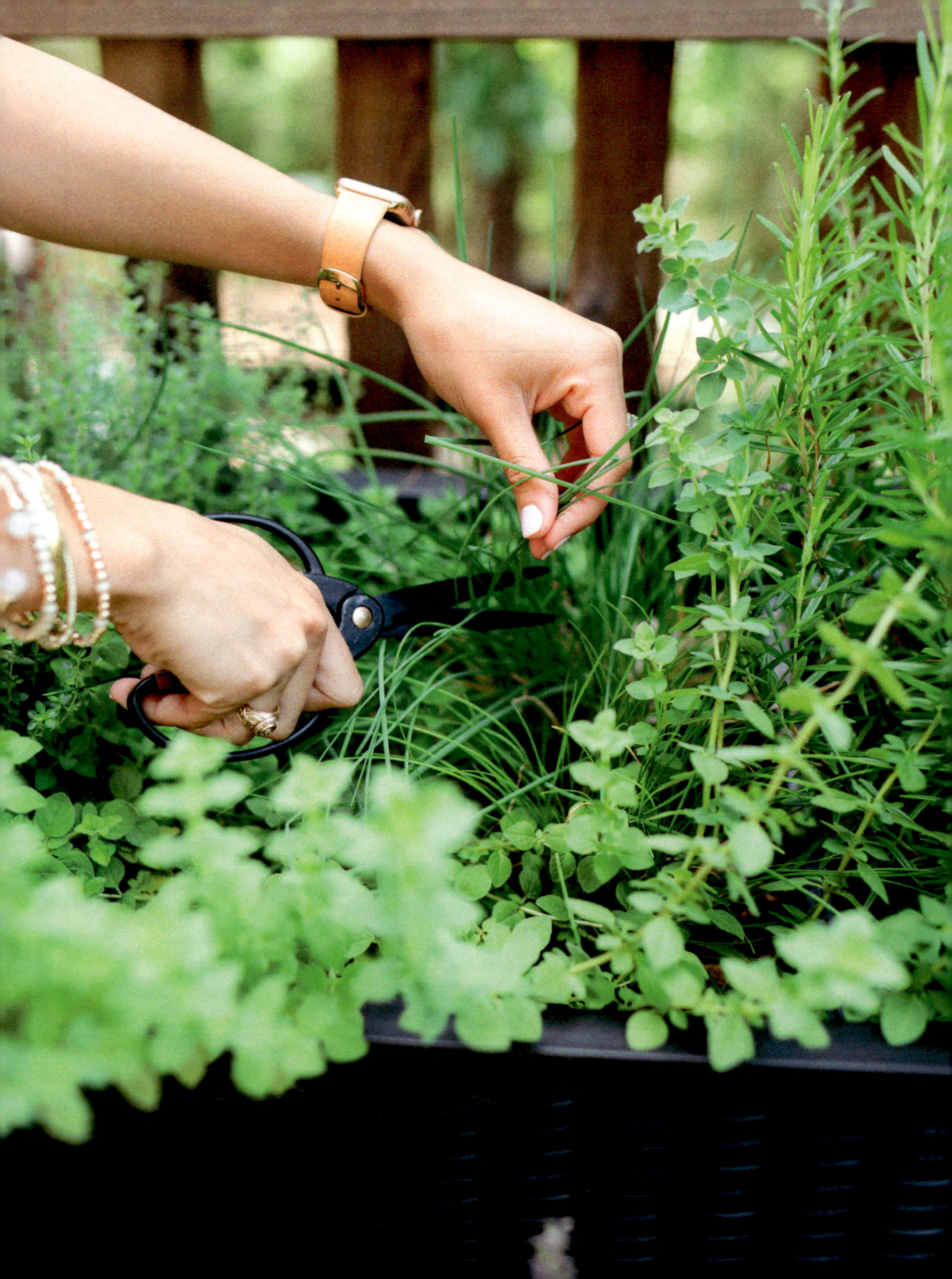

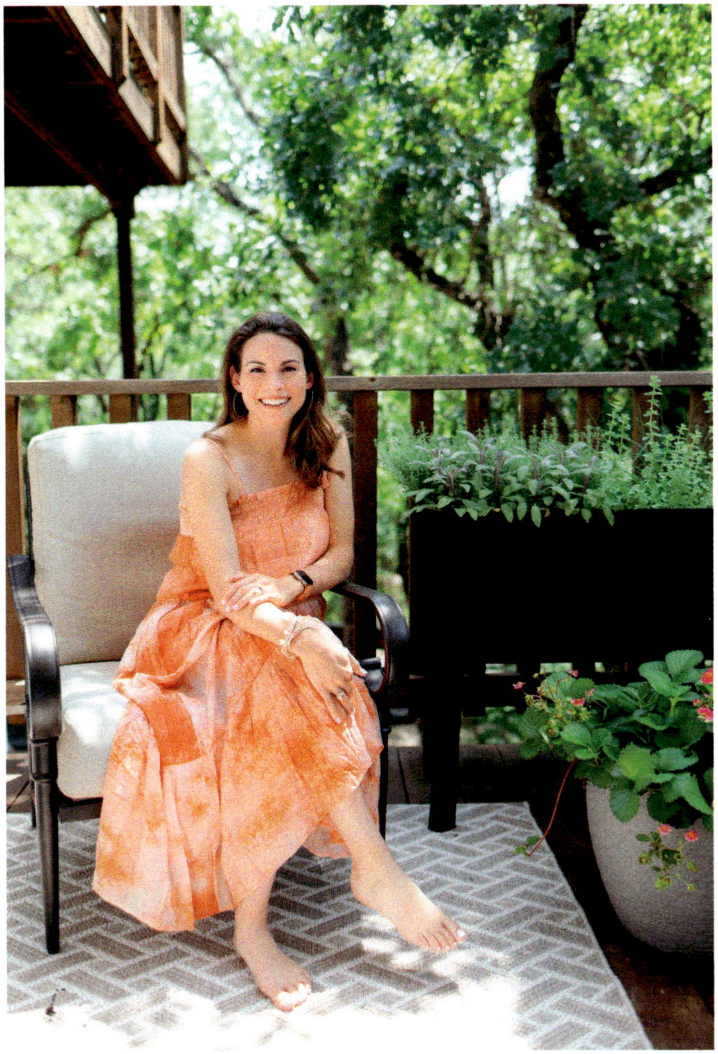

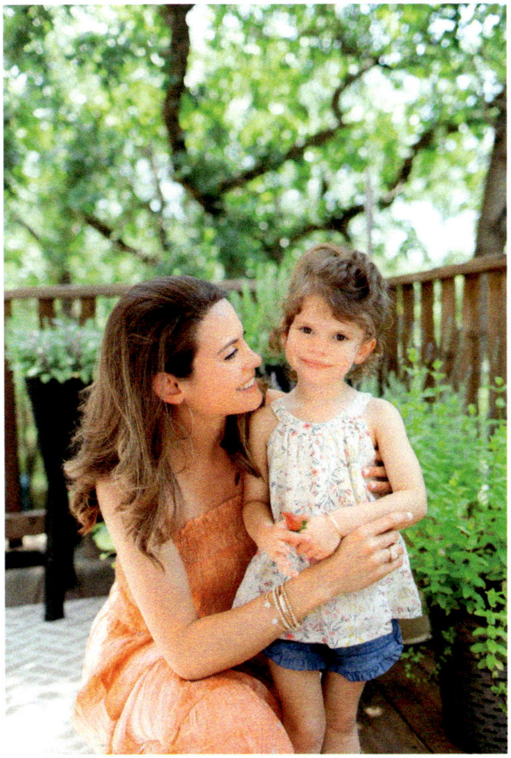

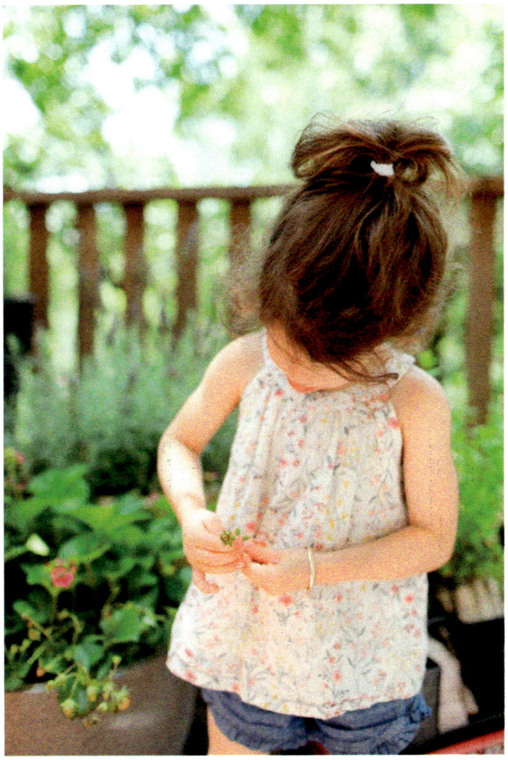

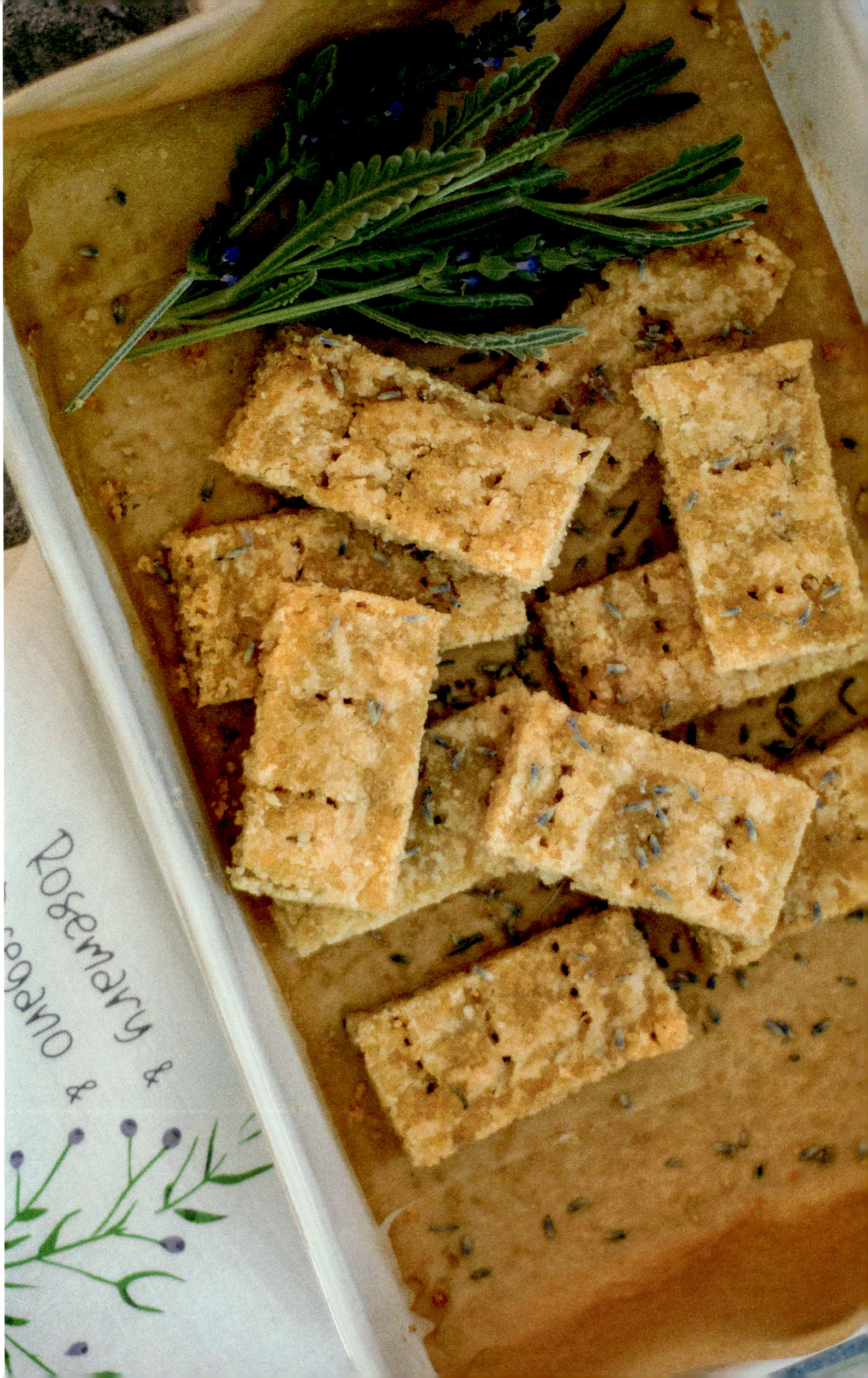

Egg Free

Nut Free

Soy Free

Mother Earth Lavender Shortbread Cookies

Lavender has been one of my favorite herbs for several years now. When Justin and I got married, the quaint bed and breakfast where we stayed (mentioned again with my breakfast bacon scones recipe) used real lavender from a local farm in all their soaps and shampoos. We even had dried lavender thrown at our wedding instead of flowers, rice, or sparklers. To this day I love diffusing lavender oil in the kitchen because the warm scent always brings back so many happy memories. Lavender has been used throughout history to help reduce anxiety, and promote relaxation, calmness, and sleep. It felt natural to put lavender in a shortbread cookie because these ingredients create such a buttery, earthy treat that's only fitting for an afternoon tea. Planning a sunday brunch, bridal or baby shower? These cookies are perfect for such an occasion.

PREP TIME: 15 minutes

INACTIVE PREP: 30 minutes to chill the dough

COOK TIME: 60 minutes

YIELDS: 16 bars

Ingredients:

¾ cup butter, softened

1 cup packed confectioner's sugar

¼ cup granulated sugar

2 tsp pure vanilla extract

1 ½ cup all purpose flour

Pinch of salt

2 tsp dried baking lavender

2-3 tbsp Turbinado sugar for sprinkling on top

Directions:

- Prepare a 9x13" baking dish with parchment paper on the bottom and up the sides (I found it better not to use cooking spray due to the oil it leaves on the bottom of the shortbread).
- Using an electric mixer, cream together the butter and both sugars until smooth. Add the vanilla extract and mix until well-combined.
- In a separate small mixing bowl, whisk together the flour, salt, and lavender.
- Add the flour mixture to the butter mixture and mix until combined. Do not over mix.
- Dump the dough into the prepared baking dish and press into the bottom of the pan. Spread the dough out evenly, using your hands to press the edges down as well.
- Sprinkle the top with turbinado sugar and chill the dough pan in the fridge for about 30 minutes.
- Preheat the oven to 300 degrees Fahrenheit while the dough is chilling.
- After the dough is chilled, bake for 60 minutes or until golden brown.
- While still warm, use a fork to puncture the shortbread with small designs. Slice the shortbread into 1"x3" bars while still warm.
- Let the shortbread cool completely before removing from the dish and transferring to a plate.

Tip:

Store either in the fridge or countertop for up to 5-6 days.

☆☆☆☆☆

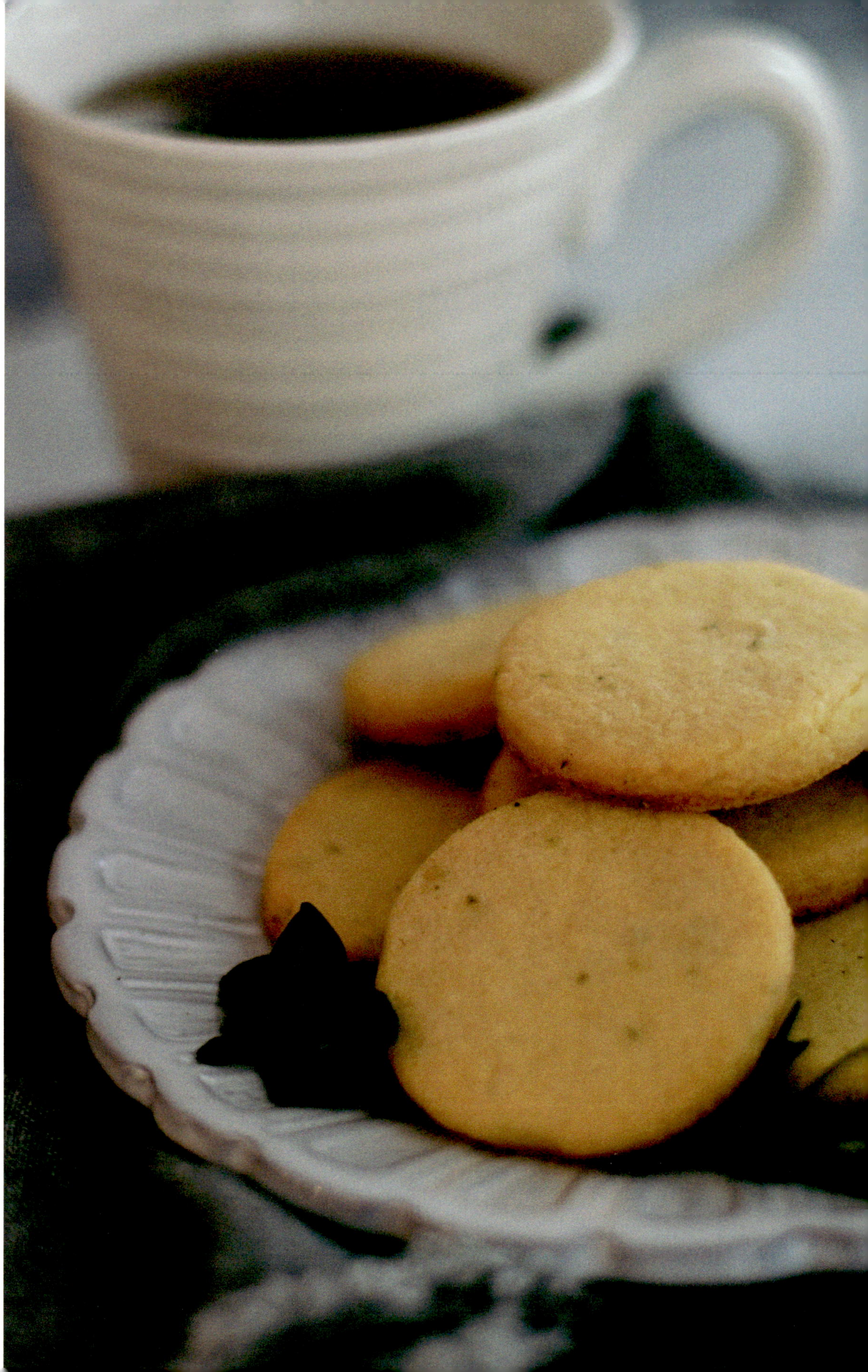

Nut Free

Soy Free

Oregano & Rosemary Butter Cookies

Perfect for a Spring or Summer weekend brunch, these butter biscuit cookies are exactly what you might think. Part biscuit, part butter cookie, the additional herbs give these cookies a boost of freshness that brings the outdoors in. They are perfect for pairing with your favorite jams such as strawberry or grape, but don't be afraid to mix it up with more exotic flavors such as strawberry jalapeno, bacon, bourbon, or even tomato jam. These are great make-ahead cookies as they can stay fresh on the countertop or can be stored in the freezer for later use. Since the recipe can make up to 36 small cookies, I recommend storing half for later last-minute brunch get-togethers.

The simple herbs, oregano & rosemary have been used throughout history for a variety of health benefits such as aiding simple ailments like indigestion and diarrhea. Oregano has also been used to help fight inflammation and improve insulin resistance in those that have type II Diabetes. Pure oregano oil has properties that seem to help with acne, dandruff, wounds, bites, and other skin conditions.

I grow both oregano and rosemary on our back porch for the sweet aroma they create and the easy access for cooking when a recipe calls for them. My sweet daughter, Emmie, loves to help water and care for my herbs almost as much as I do.

TOTAL PREP TIME: 40 mins (includes chill time)

INACTIVE PREP: 25 minutes+

COOK TIME: 15-16 minutes

YIELDS: 18 large (2.5" diameter) or 36 (2" diameter) cookies

Ingredients:

1 cup butter, softened

⅔ cup granulated sugar

2 large egg yolks, chilled

1 tsp pure vanilla extract

2 cups all purpose flour

Pinch of salt

1 ½ tsp freshly chopped oregano (can substitute for dried)

1 ½ tsp freshly chopped rosemary (can substitute for dried)

Directions:

- Preheat the oven to 350 degrees Fahrenheit. Prepare a baking sheet with parchment paper.
- In a large mixing bowl, cream together the butter and sugar until light and fluffy (about 1-2 minutes). Add the egg yolks and vanilla extract.
- In a separate mixing bowl, combine the flour, salt, and herbs.
- Combine the flour mixture with the wet ingredients and mix until well combined. Dough will be semi-dry. This is perfect!
- Place in the refrigerator to chill for at least 25 minutes (can store overnight if making these ahead of time)
- Separate the dough into 2 large portions. Using a rolling pin, roll one portion of dough out onto a lightly floured surface until about ½ inch thickness.
- Depending on desired size of cookies, (2" diameter circle or 2.5" diameter circle) and cut the dough with a cookie cutter. Use the scraps to roll out again until the dough is all used.
- Place on a baking sheet with a little room to spread. Bake for 15-16 minutes (if using 2") or 16-17 minutes (if using 2.5")

Tips:

Serve with jam and freshly steeped tea

Perfect for bridal showers, baby showers, tea parties, or brunch

Store in an airtight container for up to 1 week. Can be stored in the freezer for later use.

☆☆☆☆☆

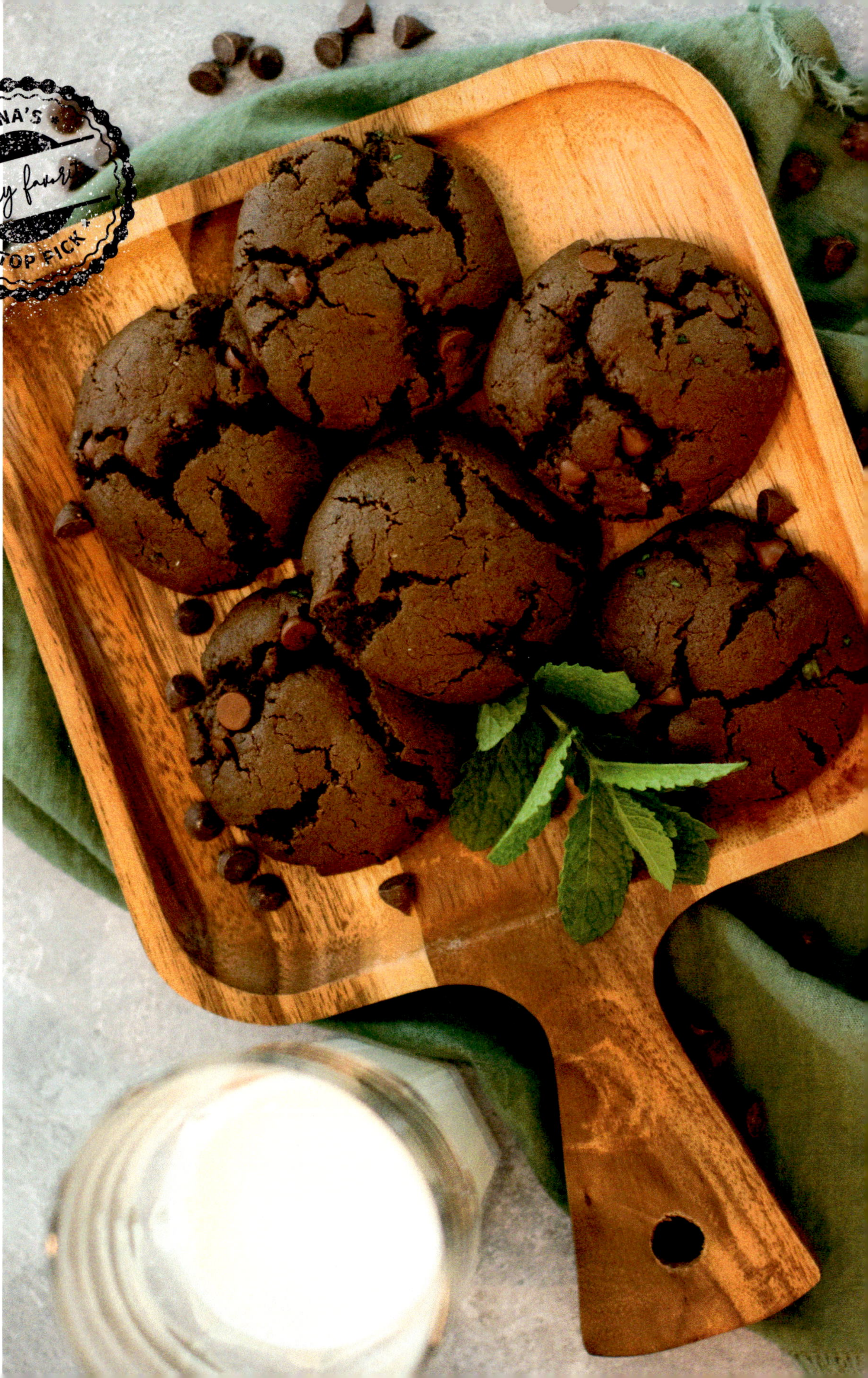

Nut Free

Soy Free

Double Chocolate Garden Mint Cookies

Peppermint has long been used as a remedy for ailments including relieving sore muscles, headaches, cold and flu, digestive problems, and even to help improve mood and appetite.

People with IBS symptoms such as bloating and abdominal pain can benefit from using peppermint's unique properties, allowing it to relieve (although not cure) the pain associated with IBS. In addition, peppermint contains a high content of menthol, which gives the sensation of cooling when ingested or used topically. Many popular desserts use peppermint as a faux fresh taste, but how many store-bought desserts use freshly picked and chopped peppermint? These cookies contain both mint extract and freshly picked/chopped peppermint to give your taste buds the REAL experience. Craving some chocolate and mint? These cookies have it all, from the rich and decadent chocolate profile to the cool and refreshing mint, these might give any popular mint chocolate cookie a run for its money.

PREP TIME: 15 minutes

COOK TIME: 11-12 minutes

YIELDS: 16 cookies

Ingredients:

1 ½ cup all purpose flour

2 tsp baking soda

Pinch of salt

½ cup naturally unsweetened 100% cocoa powder

½ cup butter, softened

½ cup granulated sugar

½ cup packed light brown sugar

1 large egg

1 tsp pure vanilla extract

1 tsp mint extract

½ cup semi-sweet chocolate chips

1 heaping tbsp freshly picked/ finely chopped mint leaves

Directions:

- Preheat the oven to 350 degrees Fahrenheit. Prepare 2 baking sheets with parchment paper.
- In a small mixing bowl, whisk together the flour, baking soda, salt, and cocoa powder. Set aside.
- In a large mixing bowl, cream together the butter and both sugars until light and fluffy (about 1-3 minutes). Add the egg, vanilla extract, and mint extract. Continue to beat until well incorporated.
- Add the dry flour mixture, ½ at a time, to the wet ingredients and continue to mix until the dough is smooth and consistent.
- Fold in the chocolate chips and chopped mint.
- Using your hands, roll the dough into 1 ½ inch balls and place it on the prepared baking sheet with room to spread.
- Bake for 11-12 minutes or until the tops begin to crack open.

Tip:

Store in an airtight container for up to 6 days.

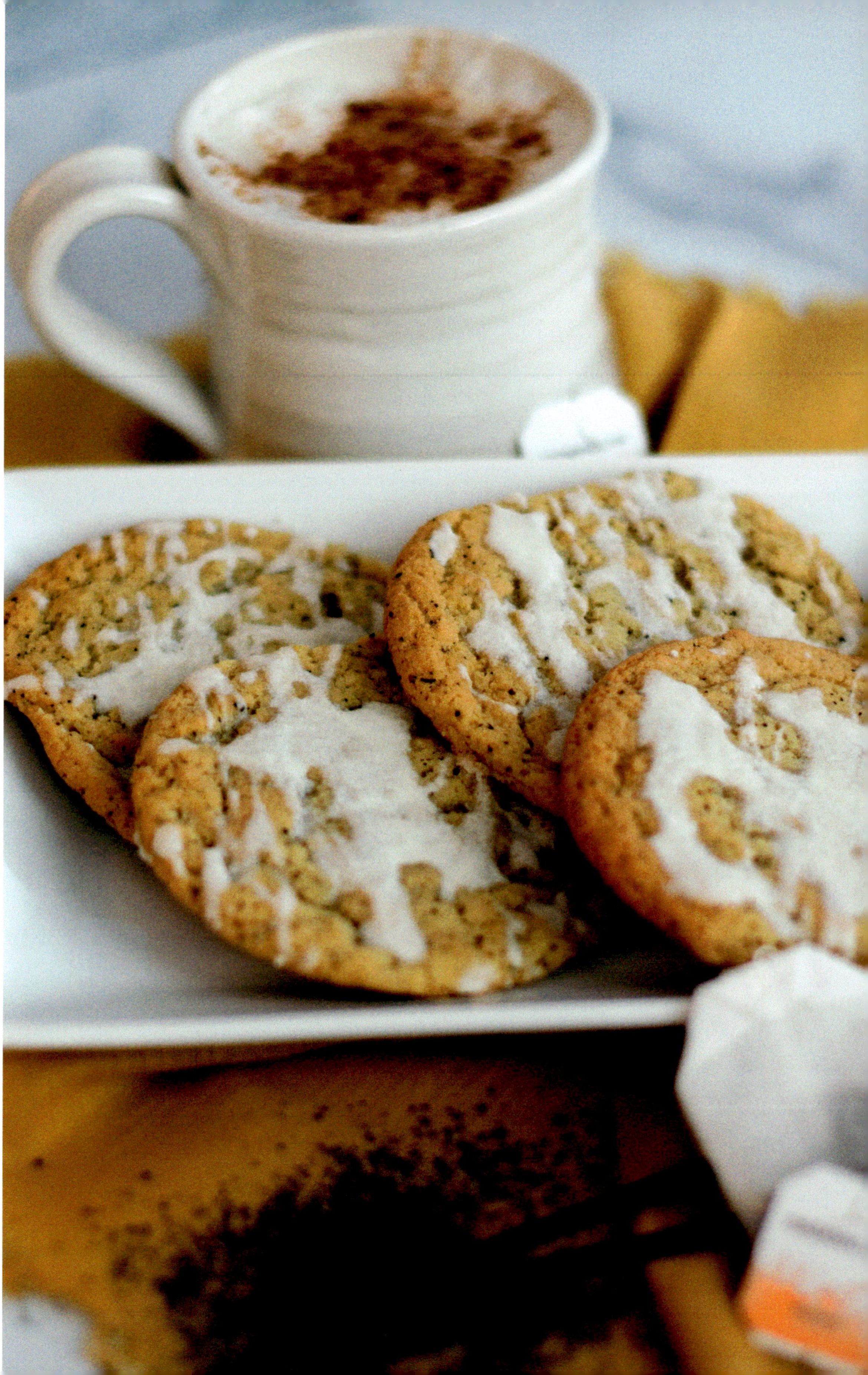

Nut Free

Soy Free

Chai Tea Latte Cookies

If you love hot chai tea as much as I do, then you'll love these classic yet sophisticated cookies that mimic the same cozy taste. Using real chai tea ingredients, the flavor is brought to life with the aroma of the warm earthy spices. The key is finding a great chai tea you already know and love. We all have our favorites but I'm partial to Tazo teas because the ingredients are wholesome. Have a favorite of your own already? Use what you have on hand and don't forget the latte glaze on top!

Chai tea contains a multitude of warming spices such as cinnamon, cardamom, ginger, anise, cloves, black pepper, nutmeg, and of course black tea. Warming spices are great for the immune system because they help fight inflammation in the body and increase blood circulation. Although you may need to eat several of these cookies to get those healthy benefits, let's just grab some hot tea and enjoy one cookie at a time...

PREP TIME: 15 minutes

COOK TIME: 12-13 minutes

YIELDS: 15 cookies

Ingredients:

COOKIE DOUGH

½ cup butter, softened

½ cup packed light brown sugar

½ cup granulated sugar

1 large egg

1 tsp pure vanilla extract

1 ½ cup all purpose flour

1 tsp baking powder

1 tsp baking soda

Pinch of salt

2 packets of chai tea
(1 Tbsp loose chai tea)

LATTE GLAZE TOPPING

¼ cup butter, softened

1 cup confectioner's sugar

1 tsp pure vanilla extract

1 tbsp milk

3 tbsp water

Directions:

- Preheat the oven to 350 degrees Fahrenheit. Prepare a baking sheet with parchment paper.
- In a large mixing bowl, cream together the butter and both sugars until light and fluffy (about 1-2 minutes). Next, add the egg and vanilla extract.
- In a separate mixing bowl, whisk together the flour, baking soda, baking powder, pinch of salt, and chai tea.
- Combine the flour mixture to the wet ingredients and mix until well combined.
- Roll into 1 inch balls (or use a 1" ice cream scoop) and place on the baking sheet with room to spread.
- Bake for 12-13 minutes or until golden brown.
- While the cookies are baking, make the glaze. Using an electric mixer, cream together the butter, sugar, vanilla, milk, and water until smooth. You may need to stop and scrape the sides a few times.
- After the cookies have completely cooled, use a whisk to drizzle the glaze over the cookies in a spatter pattern (the messier, the better!)
- Place in the fridge to let the glaze set.

Tips:

Can be stored in the fridge or on the countertop for 5-6 days.

Best served with some hot coffee, a warm latte, or freshly steeped tea.

Egg Free

Nut Free

Soy Free

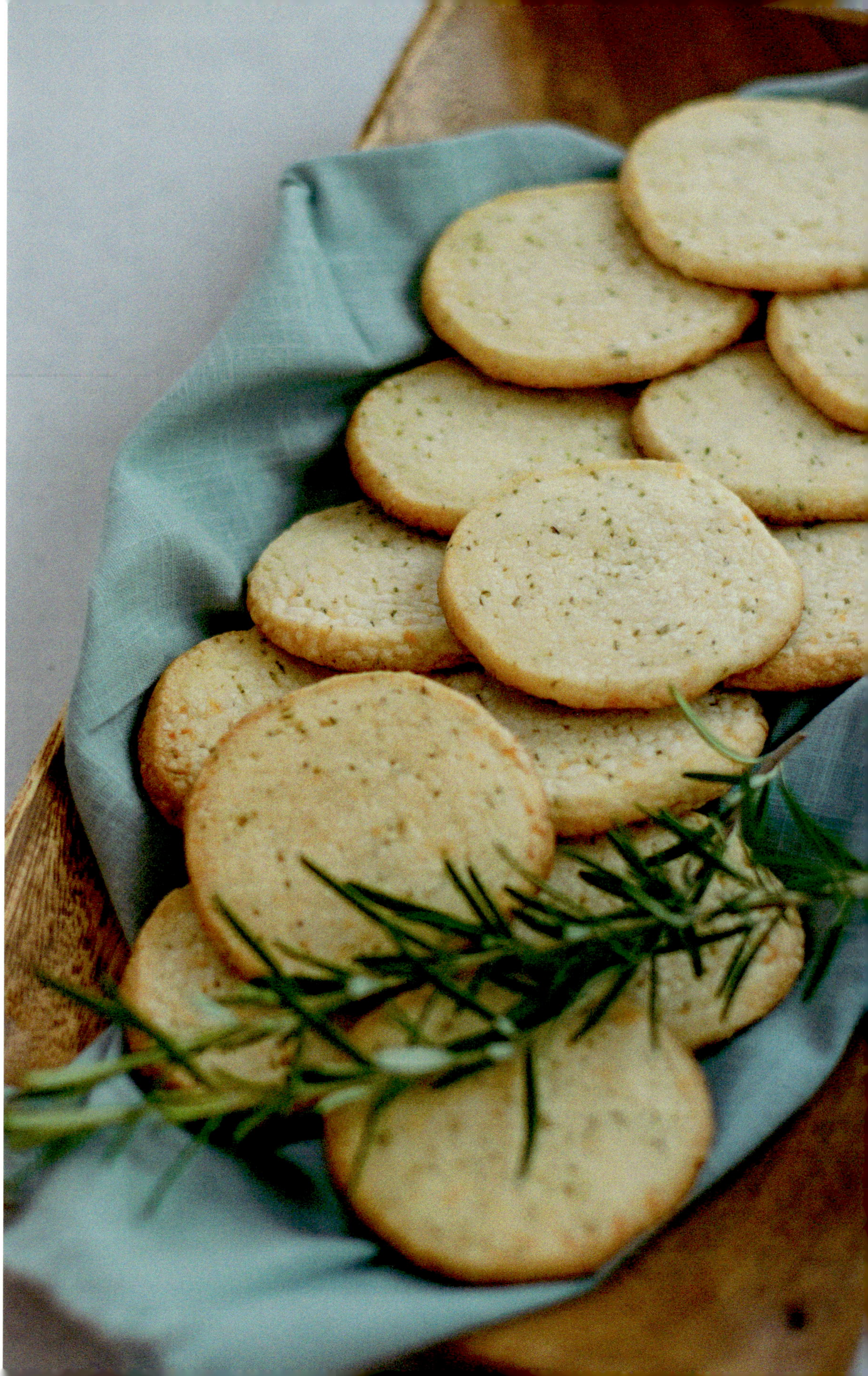

Savory Rosemary Parmesan Shortbread Cookies

There have been several medicinal uses of rosemary throughout history and old world medicine. Among many attributes, rosemary is known for its antioxidant properties that can help fight against inflammation and oxidative stress in the body. Consuming rosemary can be beneficial for the heart in increasing blood circulation and decreasing existing inflammation. Smelling rosemary has also been connected with boosting memory and cognitive function. Rosemary has always been one of my favorite herbs because of its hardy nature and warm pungent smell. I love having access to fresh rosemary on my back porch and being able to toss it in my cooking whenever I want. When baking these cookies, the aromatic smell of fresh rosemary fills the kitchen and it instantly lifts my mood. Although not a traditionally sweet cookie, these treats are wonderful by themselves or used as a soup dipper. Other ideas include topping them with some fresh bruschetta and serving as an appetizer.

TOTAL PREP TIME: 70 mins (includes chill time)

INACTIVE PREP/ CHILL TIME: 60 minutes

COOK TIME: 10-12 minutes

YIELDS: 2 ½ dozen (about 30 cookies)

Ingredients:

2 cups all purpose flour

1 cup packed confectioner's sugar

2 heaping tsp crushed dried rosemary (use fresh rosemary if available)

½ tsp salt

½ cup shredded quality parmesan cheese

1 cup butter, softened

½ tsp cold water

Directions:

- Using a large food processor, combine the flour, sugar, rosemary, salt, and parmesan cheese. Pulse together until combined.
- Add the softened butter and water and pulse again until a soft dough forms.
- Using a large piece of parchment paper, roll the dough into a log form (about 1 foot long). Wrap the dough with the remaining parchment paper and chill in the fridge for at least 1 hour. This dough can be chilled overnight if needed.
- After the dough is chilled, preheat the oven to 375 degrees Fahrenheit and prepare 2 baking sheets with parchment paper. Using a sharp knife, slice the dough log into 1/3 inch thick slices.
- Place the sliced cookies on the baking sheet and allow for slight spreading. Bake for 10-12 minutes or until the edges just begin to brown.

Tips:

Can be served with fresh tomato basil soup, with tea, or as a toast for fresh bruschetta

Perfect for bridal showers, baby showers, tea parties, or brunch

Store in an airtight container for up to 1 week. Can be stored in the freezer for later use.

☆☆☆☆☆

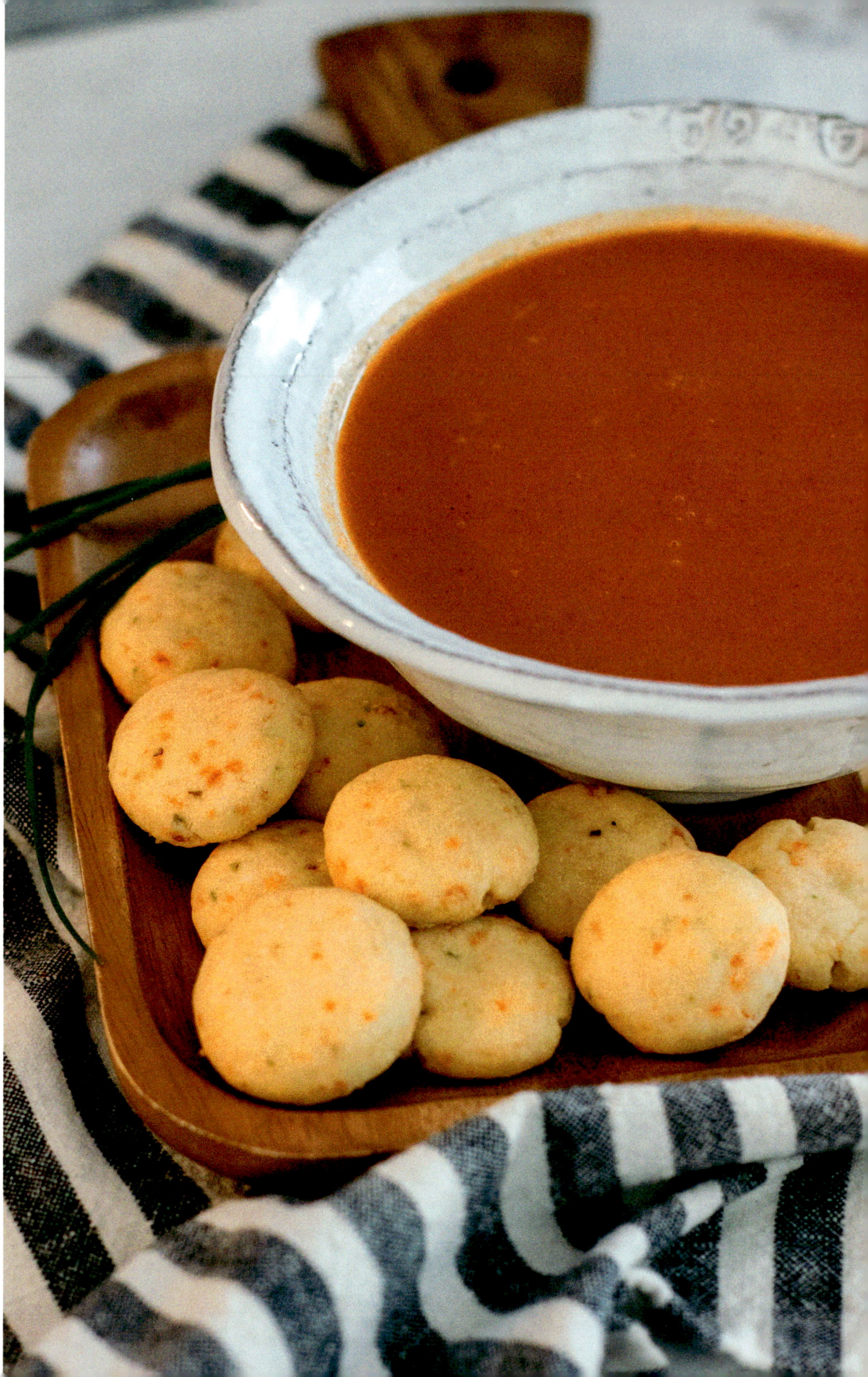

Sugar Free

Egg Free

Nut Free

Soy Free

Mini Cheddar and Chive Crackers

These crackers put a different spin on the word *cookie*, yet I wanted to include these tasty, savory bites because they are so easy to make. They pair incredibly well with hot soup, or as a midday snack alongside your favorite hummus dip. Emmie loved munching on them alongside her lunch and dinner meals, which gave her taste buds a chance to explore some unique flavors.

Chives are part of the Allium family of vegetables, also home to garlic and onions. Chives are frequently mistaken for green onions and scallions. Although they are different types of produce they can usually be used interchangeably. Chives contain several health benefits, although one would need to consume a large quantity of onions before absorbing any beneficial quantities of vitamins such as vitamin K, folate, lutein, and zeaxanthin.

TOTAL PREP TIME: 15 minutes

COOK TIME: 12-13 minutes

YIELDS: 50+ crackers

Ingredients:

2 cups all purpose flour

1 cup shredded sharp cheddar cheese

½ tsp crushed red pepper flakes

1 tbsp fresh chopped chives (or fresh green onions)

1 tsp salt

1 cup butter, softened

Directions:

- Preheat the oven to 375 degrees Fahrenheit and prepare 2 baking sheets with parchment paper.
- Using a large food processor, combine the flour, cheddar cheese, red pepper, chives, and salt. Pulse together until combined.
- Add the softened butter and pulse again until a soft dough forms.
- Using a teaspoon or size #100 ice cream scoop, begin scooping the dough out and rolling together with your hands. Place on the prepared baking sheet and lightly smash down with your fingers or spatula until it forms a disc shape. Crackers will not spread much, so place them close together while baking to save room.
- Bake for 12-13 minutes or until the cheddar cheese begins to turn slightly orange.

Tips:

Serve with warm soup or alongside any savory meal for an added cheesy crunch. Great for kids snacks paired with fresh veggies or dip of choice (hummus, ranch, etc)

Store in an airtight container for up to 1 week

☆☆☆☆☆

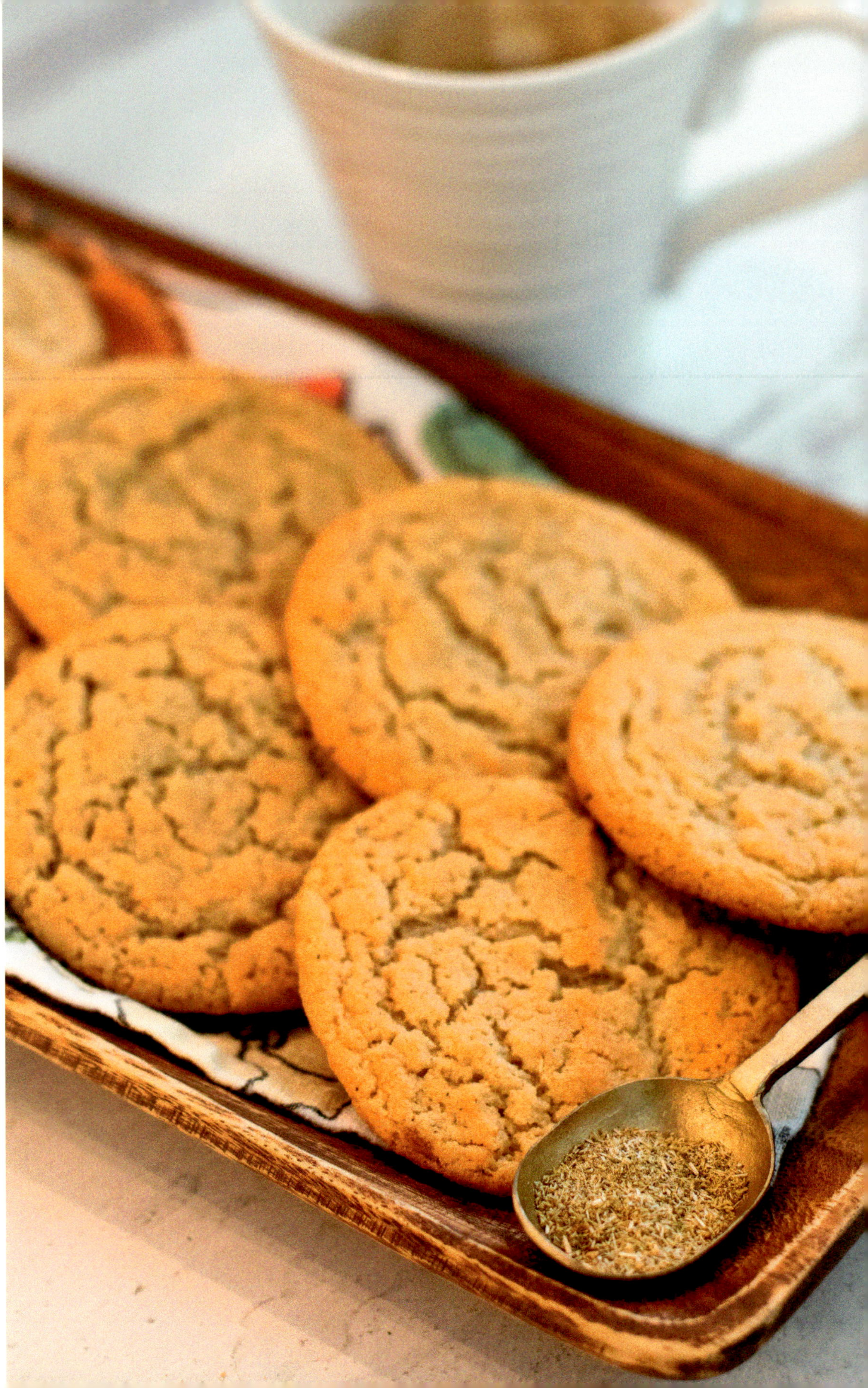

Nut Free

Soy Free

Simply Sweet Chamomile Tea Cookies

Chamomile in itself is a dainty yet beautiful wildflower. I love the simple charm of its tiny white petals and sunshine-yellow middle. Besides chamomile's delicate features, it has long been used to help promote calmness and soothe the nervous system. I like to drink chamomile tea in the evenings when I'm restless; it's like a warm hug in a mug and leads to a refreshing night's sleep. Its medicinal properties have also been used to ease anxiety, pain, and digestive woes. Gentle enough for even your toddlers, chamomile is a great choice when they need a little extra help soothing--think of Peter Rabbit's wise mother who served him chamomile tea after escaping Mr. McGregor's garden.

TOTAL PREP TIME: 15 minutes

COOK TIME: 10-12 minutes

YIELDS: 16-17 cookies

Ingredients:

½ cup butter, softened

½ cup packed light brown sugar

½ cup granulated sugar

1 large egg

1 tsp pure vanilla extract

1 ½ cup all purpose flour

1 tsp baking powder

1 tsp baking soda

Pinch of salt

2 packets of cchamomile tea (1 Tbsp loose chamomile tea)

Directions:

- Preheat the oven to 350 degrees Fahrenheit. Prepare 2 baking sheets with parchment paper.
- In a large mixing bowl, cream together the butter and both sugars until light and fluffy (about 2-3 minutes). Add the egg and vanilla extract.
- In a separate mixing bowl, whisk together the flour, baking soda, baking powder, pinch of salt, and camomile tea.
- Combine the flour mixture to the wet ingredients and mix until well combined.
- Roll into 1 inch balls (or use a 1" ice cream scoop) and place on the baking sheet with room to spread.
- Bake for 10-12 minutes or until golden brown.

Tips:

Store in an airtight container for up to 1 week.

Best served with some hot coffee, a warm latte, or freshly steeped tea.

☆☆☆☆☆

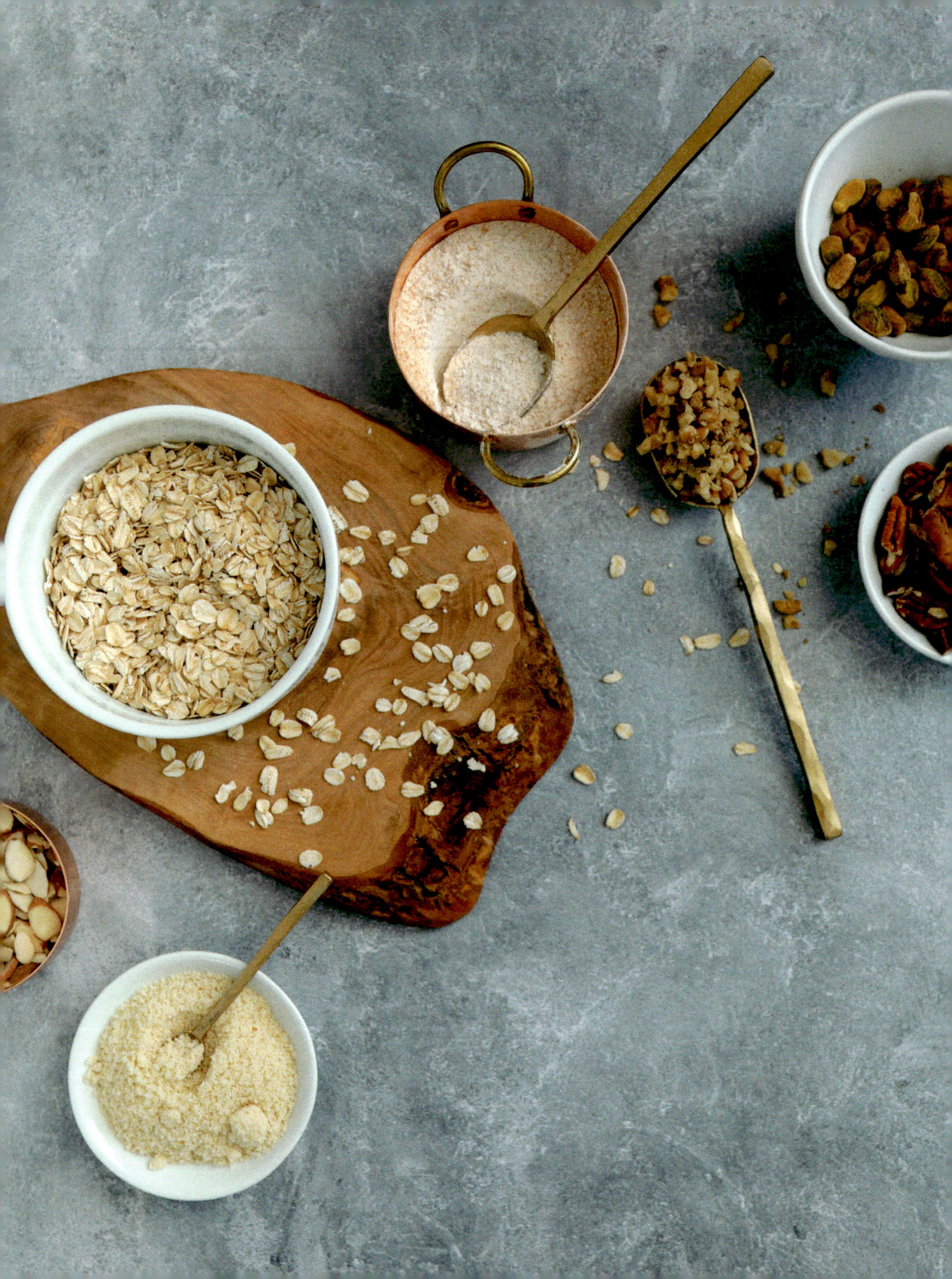

Gluten Free Favorites

- Crunchy Almond Butter Cookies
- Granola Bar Cookies
- Chocolate Avocado Cookies
- Steph's Oatmeal Carrot Cake Cookies
- Pumpkin Chocolate Chip Cookies
- Emmie's Mini PB&J Cookies
- Simple Pecan Sandies *(Steph's Pick)*
- Steph's Antioxidant Chocolate Bark *(Steph's Pick)*
- Chunky Monkey Banana Pudding Cookies
- Fresh Lemon Curd Cookies *(LFD's Pick)*
- Candied Orange Ginger Cookies
- No Bake Figgy Pops
- Chewy Orange Almond Cookies
- Nutty n' Pink Whoopies

Gluten-Free Flours and Nuts

1:1 Gluten Free Flour

Brand: Bob's Red Mill

Combination of gluten free flours, starches, and xanthan gum.The texture is very similar and comparable to that of regular flour.

Contains only a slight gritty texture in baked goods, this flour's taste is comparable to that of regular, all-purpose flour.

Almonds

Almonds can be eaten with or without the skin and contain a smooth nutty taste profile.

They are rich in unsaturated fat and contain vitamin E, calcium, zinc, protein, and fiber.

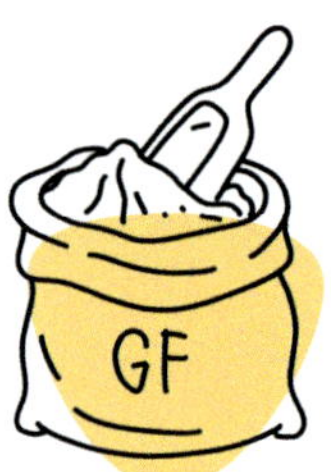

Almond Flour

Finely ground almonds made with blanched almonds that have been previously skinned. Baked goods with almond flour tend to be soft and delicate.

Nutty, slightly sweet in flavor when used in baking.

Ground Flax Seeds

Not as finely ground as a traditional flour, ground flaxseeds have a mild woody & nutty flavor that can be hidden in many baked goods.

Great source of dietary fiber (both soluble and insoluble).

Ground Oatmeal Flour

Homemade oat flour is the process of finely grinding up old fashioned oats in a food processor until it resembles a soft, flour-like texture.

Earthy in taste, oatmeal flour can also become very dense when cooked/baked. Oatmeal flour can replace regular all-purpose flour in a 1:1 ratio by weight, not volume.

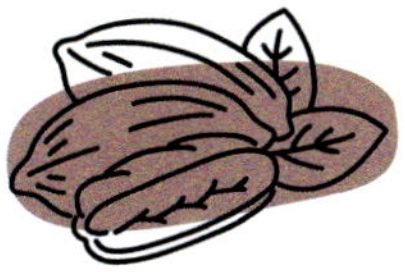

Pecans

Slightly sweet with a nutty and buttery flavor, pecans are the most popular nut to bake with. They are versatile and pair well with almost any dessert.
They contain a good source of calcium, magnesium, potassium, and are rich in healthy monounsaturated fats.

Pistachios

The high fat content allows for a meaty crunch and a light, buttery, almost salty nut flavor.
Excellent source of protein, antioxidants, fiber, and vitamin B6. Diet rich in pistachios can help to manage blood sugar, improve heart health, gut health, and eye health.

Quick Oats

Rolled oats that have gone through the process of partial steam cooking and then rolled even thinner than traditional old fashioned rolled oats. When cooked/baked these oats are soft and mushy.
The taste is mild and much like that of traditional rolled oats.

Rolled Oats

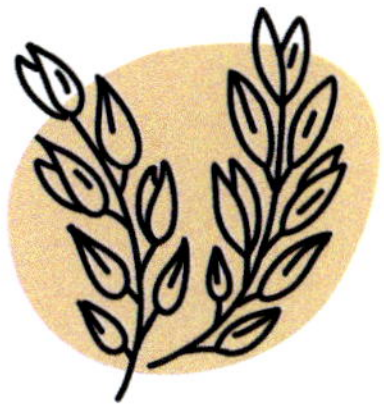

Oat grains that have been partially steamed and rolled through a flattening process. When cooked/baked they exhibit a sticky, and thick texture.
Much like quick oats, old fashioned oats are mild with a slight earthy, nutty taste.

Walnuts

Slightly bitter in taste, walnuts are also earthy. The taste and tannin profile complements sweet foods such as bananas, caramel, and maple syrup as well as high-fat ingredients like butter, cheese, and rich milk chocolate.
Walnuts are high in omega-3 fatty acids as well as protein, fiber, and magnesium.

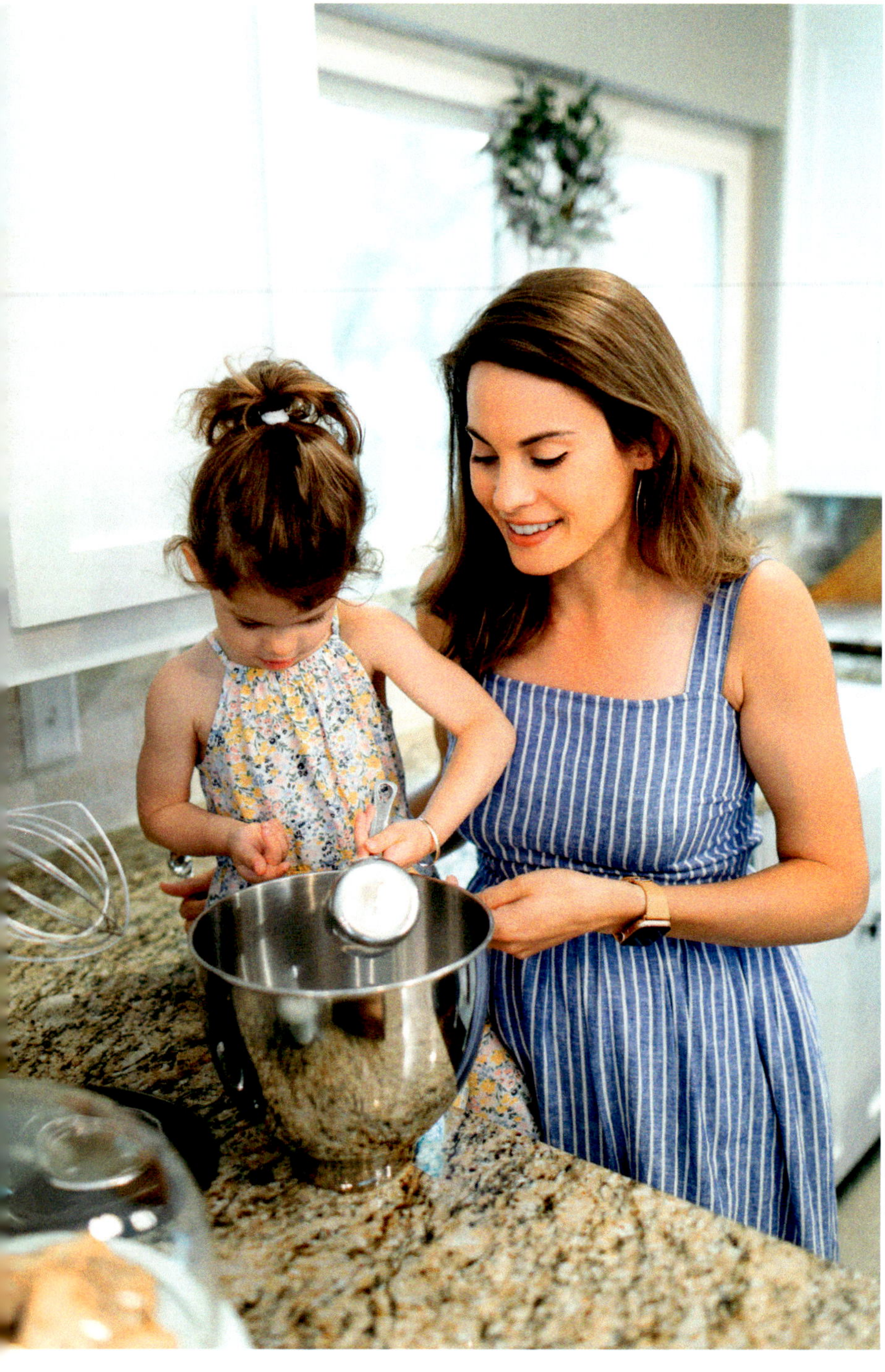
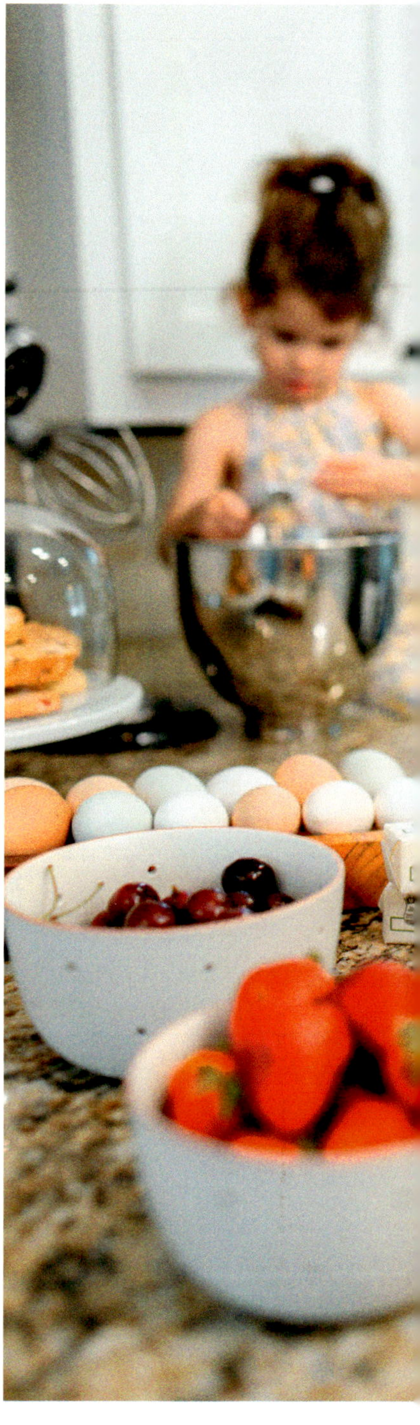

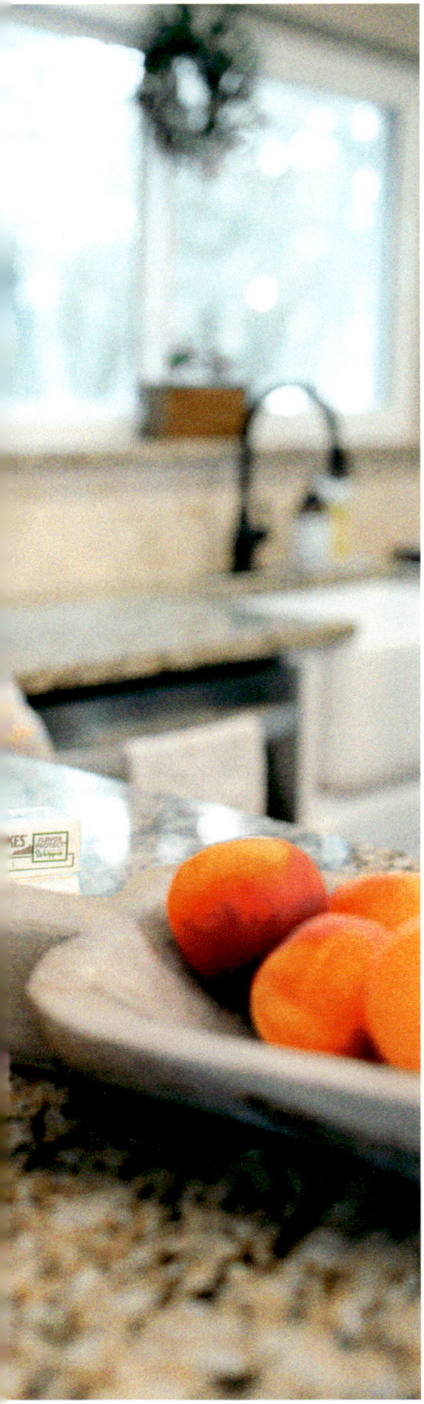

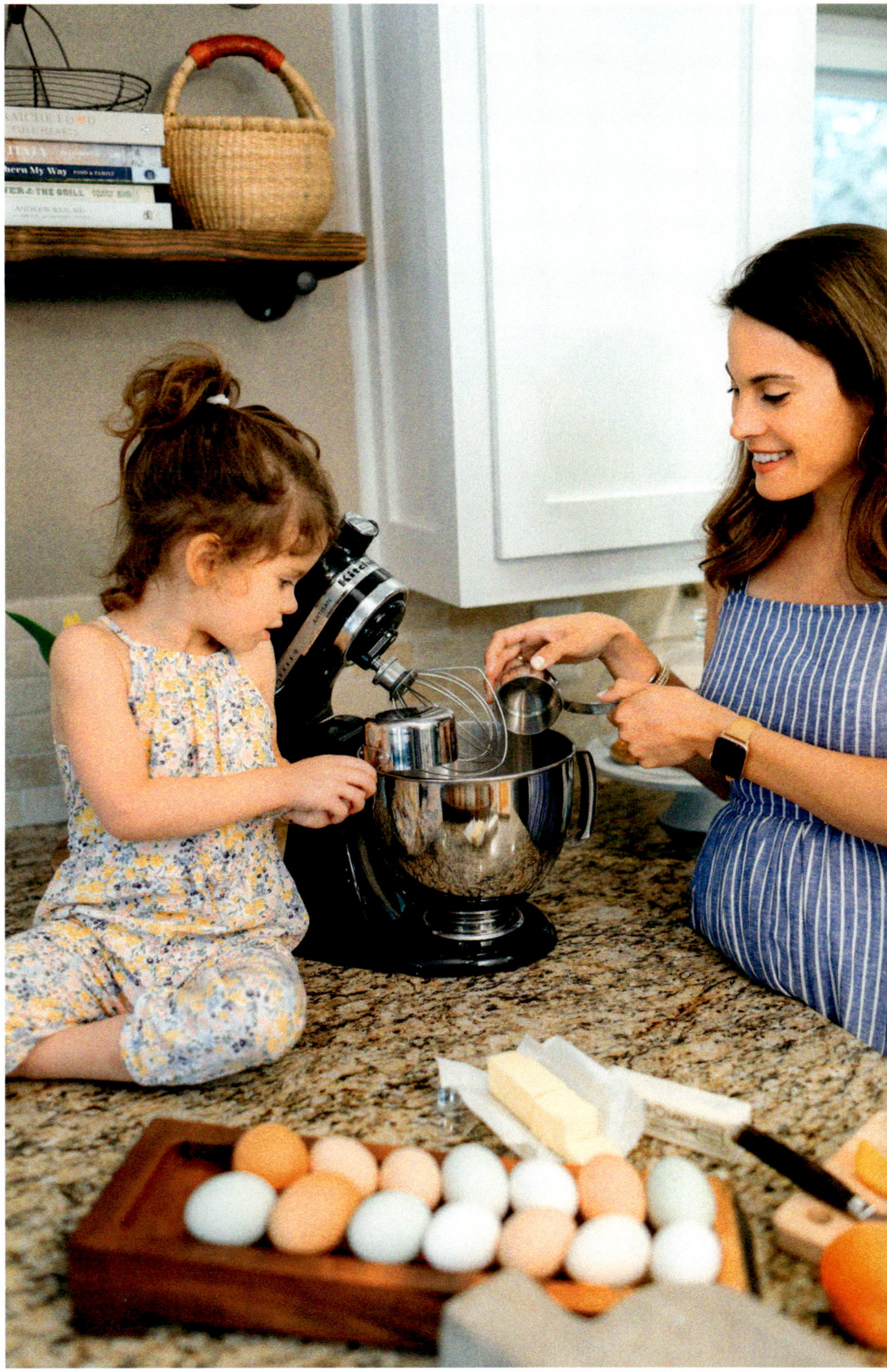

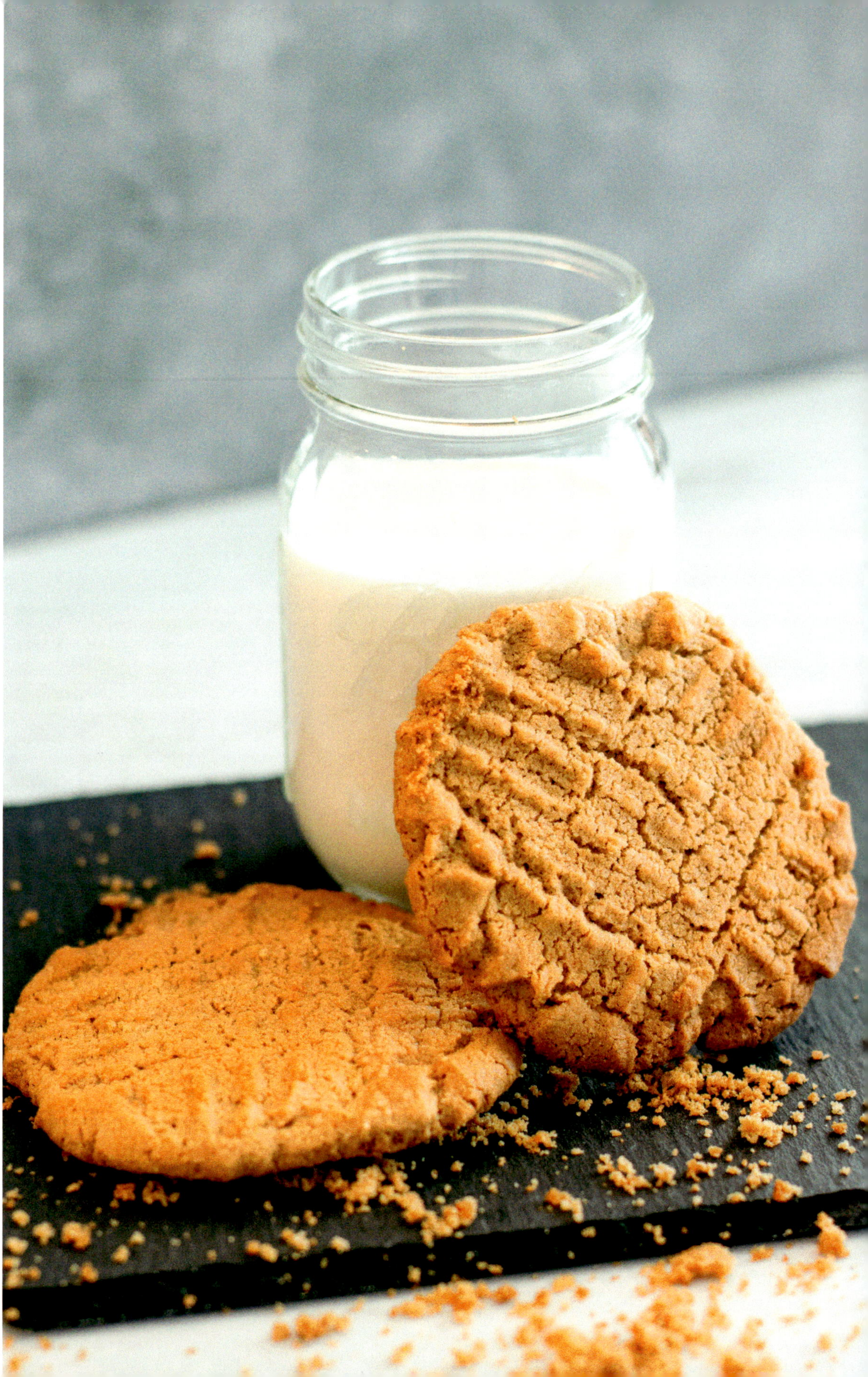

Gluten Free

Soy Free

GF Crunchy Almond Butter Cookies

These cookies were made almost by accident. I was originally going for a soft, gooey, almond butter cookie, yet these crumbly decadent treats came out instead. I was on the fence between throwing them out and starting over again when Justin tried them and was hooked from the first bite. He then took them to his co-workers who devoured them in a few short hours. To my dismay, everybody LOVED them and were asking for more! So here we are: the original munchy crunchy almond butter cookie remains. Grab a glass of cold milk and get ready to dunk!
Almonds are excellent sources of vitamin E, magnesium, and heart-healthy monounsaturated fats.

OVERALL PREP TIME: 30 minutes

CHILL TIME: 15-20 minutes

COOK TIME: 14-15 minutes

YIELDS: 18-19 cookies

Ingredients:

½ cup butter, softened

1 cup creamy style almond butter (I love MaraNatha™)

1 cup packed light brown sugar

1 large egg

1 tsp pure vanilla extract

1 cup 1:1 gluten-free flour

1 tsp baking soda

Pinch of salt

Directions:

- Preheat the oven to 350 degrees Fahrenheit. Prepare a baking sheet with parchment paper.
- In a large mixing bowl, mix together the softened butter and almond butter with a spoon. Next, add the brown sugar and continue to mix. Lastly, add the egg and vanilla and mix until combined.
- In a separate mixing bowl, combine the gluten-free flour, baking soda, and salt. Mix well.
- Pour the dry mixture into the almond butter mixture using a spatula. Mix until well-combined.
- Chill dough for about 15-20 minutes in the refrigerator.
- Using a Scoop #40 (1½ size), spoon out the batter. Then, using your hands, continue to make individual round balls and place them on the baking sheet with ample room to spread.
- Once dough balls are formed, press down into the dough using a fork to create a 'criss-cross' shape.
- Bake for 14-15 minutes or until lightly browned on the edges.

Tips:

Store in an airtight container for up to 6 days.

If looking for a softer cookie texture, don't press down on the cookies or simply bake less amount of time (13 minutes).

Can be made with regular all-purpose flour in place of gluten-free flour; use 1:1 ratio.

☆☆☆☆☆

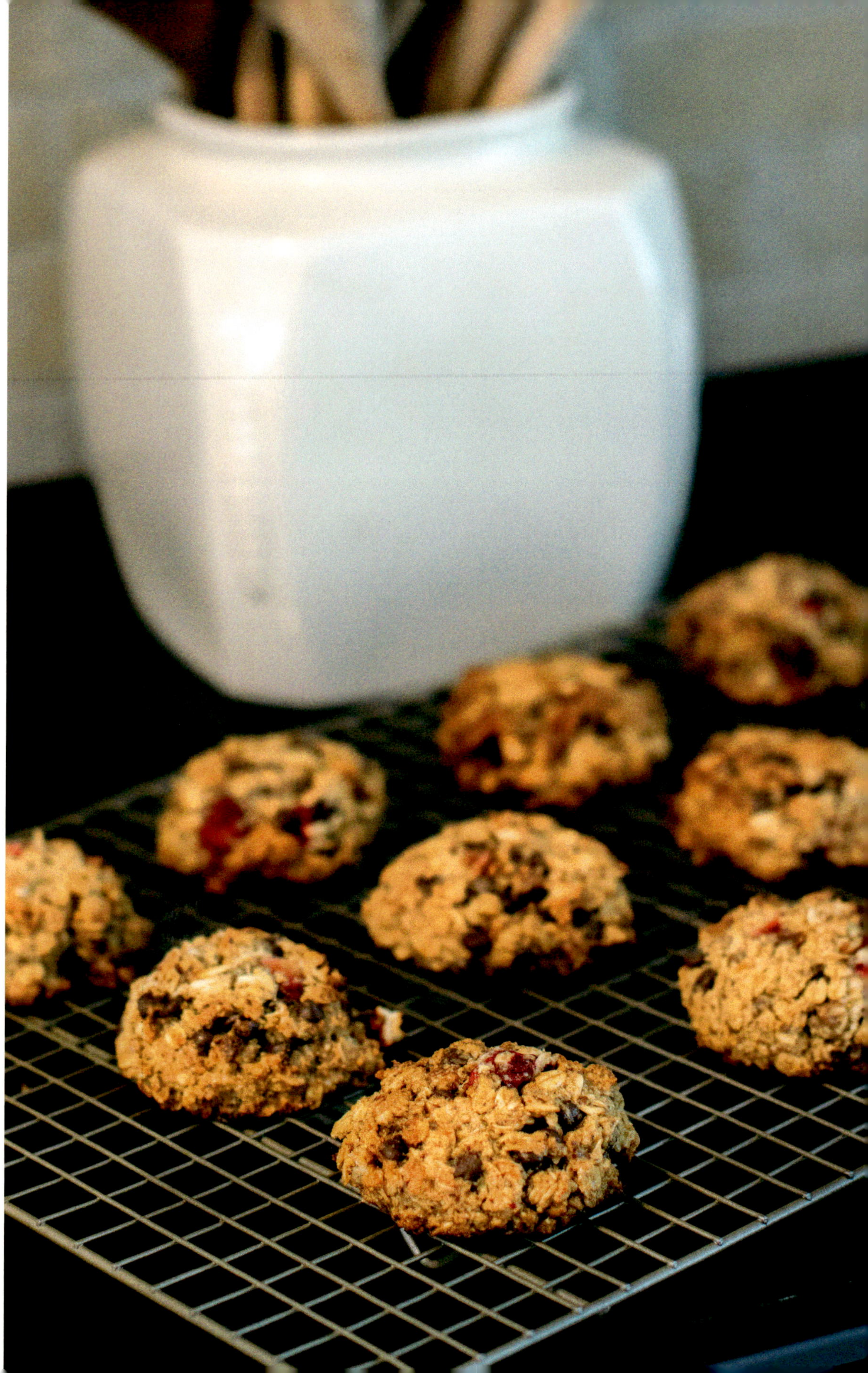

Gluten Free

Soy Free

GF Granola Bar Cookies

One of my favorite cookies to make ahead of time, freeze for later or use throughout the week as a healthy snack alternative. Yes, a cookie can be a healthy snack! Although not quite a cookie, not quite a granola bar, these little guys are mighty in flavor and nutrient power. I love that they contain minimal refined sugar, remain gluten free, & contain high amounts of fiber, healthy fats, and vitamin C! Personally, I think the cranberries create such a sweet burst of flavor in every bite, together with the chocolate chips, it's a perfect duo!

PREP TIME: 15 minutes

COOK TIME: 15-17 minutes

YIELDS: 12 cookies

Ingredients:

1 large egg

4 tbsp butter, softened

¼ cup honey

½ cup fig jam

2 tbsp packed light brown sugar

2 cups old fashioned rolled oats

1 cup almond flour

⅓ cup ground flax seeds

Pinch of salt

¾ cup frozen cranberries

½ cup coarsely chopped pecans

½ cup semi-sweet mini chocolate chips

Directions:

- Preheat the oven to 375 degrees Fahrenheit. Prepare a baking sheet with parchment paper.
- In a large mixing bowl, whisk together the egg, butter, honey, fig jam, and brown sugar.
- In a separate mixing bowl, combine the rolled oats, almond flour, ground flax seeds, and salt.
- Pour the granola mixture in the wet ingredients. Then using a spatula, mix until well combined.
- Using a Scoop #40 (1½ size), spoon out the batter and drop onto the prepared baking sheet. The batter will want to separate slightly; using your hands, mold the cookies back together and lightly flatten the balls.
- Bake for 15-17 minutes or until lightly browned on the edges.

Tips:

Store in the refrigerator for up to 6 days.

Best served re-warmed for 10 seconds in the microwave.

Great snack to bring along your adventures and a great option for kids!

☆☆☆☆☆

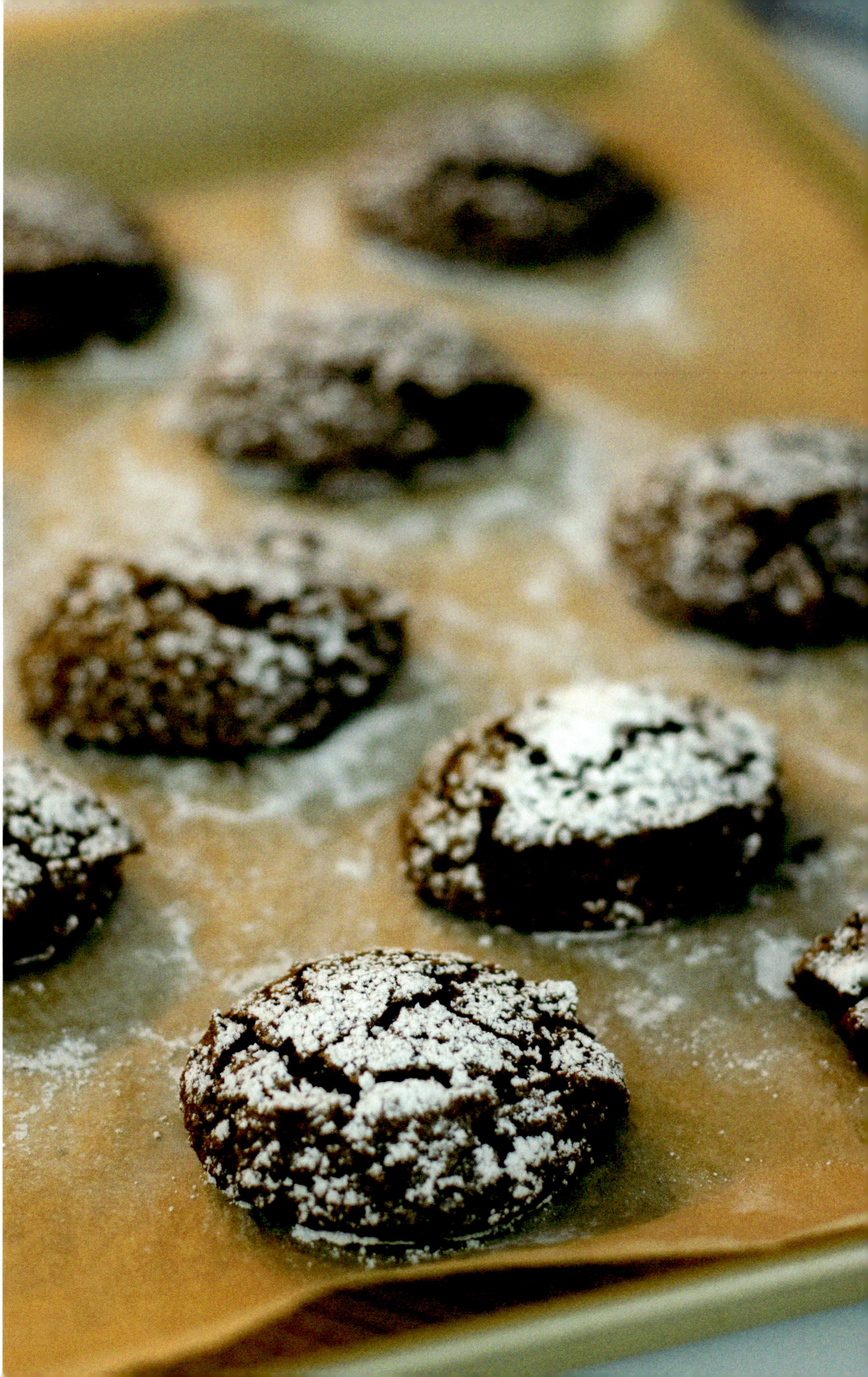

Nut Free

Dairy Free

Gluten Free

Soy Free

GF Chocolate Avocado Cookies

We all know that avocados are good for us. In fact, my interest in the health benefits of avocados is what kick-started my nutrition blog in 2015. Avocado toast for breakfast, avocado slices with lunch, avocado dip at dinner, but putting avocados in a cookie? You've got to be kidding, right? Absolutely not.

The avocado is loaded with healthy monounsaturated fats, which give these cookies an incredibly moist texture. Not to mention all the other health benefits like B vitamins, fiber, folic acid, lutein, potassium, and vitamin E. Still don't trust me? I implore you to try them; they got a thumbs up from my entire family, including the cookie connoisseur, Justin.

PREP TIME: 15 minutes

COOK TIME: 17-19 minutes

YIELDS: 15 cookies

Ingredients:

1 medium-sized avocado, mashed

1 cup granulated sugar

2 large eggs

1 tbsp vanilla extract

1 ½ cup almond flour

½ cup 100% natural cocoa powder

1 heaping tsp baking powder

Pinch of salt

½ cup confectioners sugar

Directions:

- Preheat the oven to 350 degrees Fahrenheit. Prepare a baking sheet with parchment paper.
- In a large mixing bowl, cream together the mashed avocado and sugar until a light green foamy mixture appears (about 1 minute). Add the eggs, and vanilla and continue to beat until incorporated.
- In a separate mixing bowl, combine the almond flour, cocoa powder, baking powder, and pinch of salt.
- Combine the flour mixture with the wet ingredients and mix until well combined.
- Using a Scoop #100 (1 inch size) or a Scoop #40 (1½ inches size), spoon out the batter and drop it onto the prepared baking sheet. Batter will be fairly loose and liquidy. Allow for slight expansion when cooking.
- Using a sifter or a small strainer, lightly dust the cookies with the confectioner's sugar before baking.
- Bake for 17-19 minutes

Tip:

Store in an airtight container for up to 2 days on the counter, or place in the refrigerator for up to 6 days.

☆☆☆☆☆

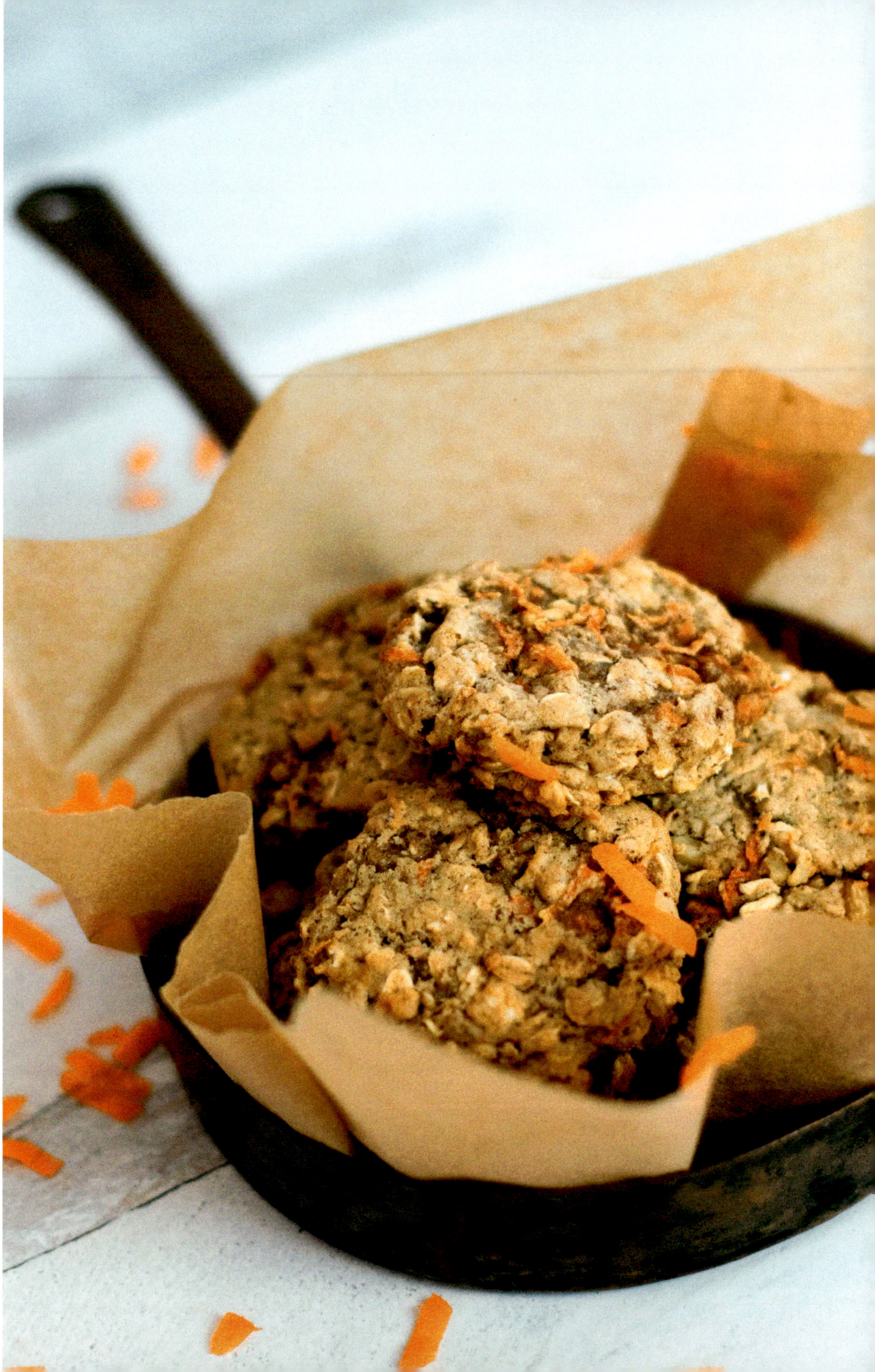

Dairy Free

Gluten Free

Egg Free

Soy Free

GF Steph's Oatmeal Carrot Cake Cookies

Let me share a bit of my personal history with you. When I was in college, I was on the World Famous Kilgore College Rangerette Drill Team in East Texas (if you don't know who this team is, I recommend looking them up for your sake). Our hours were demanding, and our training was extensive. I was young and in such great shape that my friends and I would eat a whole sheet cake of dense carrot cake with cream cheese frosting, and I swear we never gained a pound. I still think of those glory days when I see a carrot cake listed on the dessert menu or when I stroll past a bakery and smell the fresh warm spices baking. After being diagnosed with Hashimoto's and taking gluten out of my diet, there were certain indulgences I was keen on making allergen-free. So many of us have dietary restrictions or know someone else who is restricted. Baking for them is always a challenge, but I wanted to include a few specialty recipes that could be enjoyed by everybody, regardless of their dietary lifestyle.

OVERALL PREP TIME: 25 minutes

COOK TIME: 12-13 minutes

YIELDS: 20 Cookies

Ingredients:

1 mashed banana (or ½ cup butter, softened)
½ cup granulated sugar
½ cup packed light brown sugar
1 tbsp oil (avocado, canola, or coconut- omit if using butter/eggs)
1 tbsp egg replacer mixture (1 tbsp egg replacer + 2 tbsp water, mixed well -or 1 large egg)
1 tsp pure vanilla extract
1 cup 1:1 gluten-free flour
1 tsp baking soda
1 tsp baking powder
½ tsp ground cinnamon
½ tsp ground nutmeg
Pinch of salt
1 ½ cup old fashioned rolled oats
½ cup chopped walnuts
½ cup finely grated carrots

Optional: Cream Cheese Frosting (GF, SF, EF, NF)
3 tbsp butter, softened
¾ cup confectioner's sugar
2 tbsp cream cheese, softened
½ tsp pure vanilla extract
Small pinch of salt

Directions:

- Preheat the oven to 350 degrees Fahrenheit. Prepare 2 baking sheets with parchment paper.
- In a small mixing bowl, whisk together the gluten-free flour, baking soda, baking powder, cinnamon, nutmeg, and salt. Set aside.
- In a separate mixing bowl using an electric mixer, cream together the mashed banana and both sugars until light in color and smooth texture is formed (about 1-3 minutes). Add the oil, pre-mixed egg replacer, vanilla and continue to mix until well combined.
- Add the dry flour mixture, half at a time, to the wet ingredients and continue to mix until the dough is smooth and consistent.
- Add the rolled oats and continue to mix until just combined, do not overmix.
- Fold in the chopped walnuts and carrots.
- Using a Scoop #40 (1 ½ inches size), measure and place each cookie on the prepared baking sheet with very little room to spread.
- Bake for 10 minutes. While still in the oven, using a spatula, gently press the cookies flat and return to baking for another 2 minutes.

***If using the optional cream cheese frosting**

- Begin making the frosting while the cookies are baking.
- Place all frosting ingredients in a small mixing bowl and whisk together until smooth and creamy. You may also use an electric mixer to save time and arm power.
- Let cookies cool completely before frosting the tops.

Tips:

Store in the fridge for up to 6 days.
Can also substitute the cream cheese frosting for my coconut cream frosting (dairy free) see pumpkin spice snickerdoodle for recipe.

☆☆☆☆☆

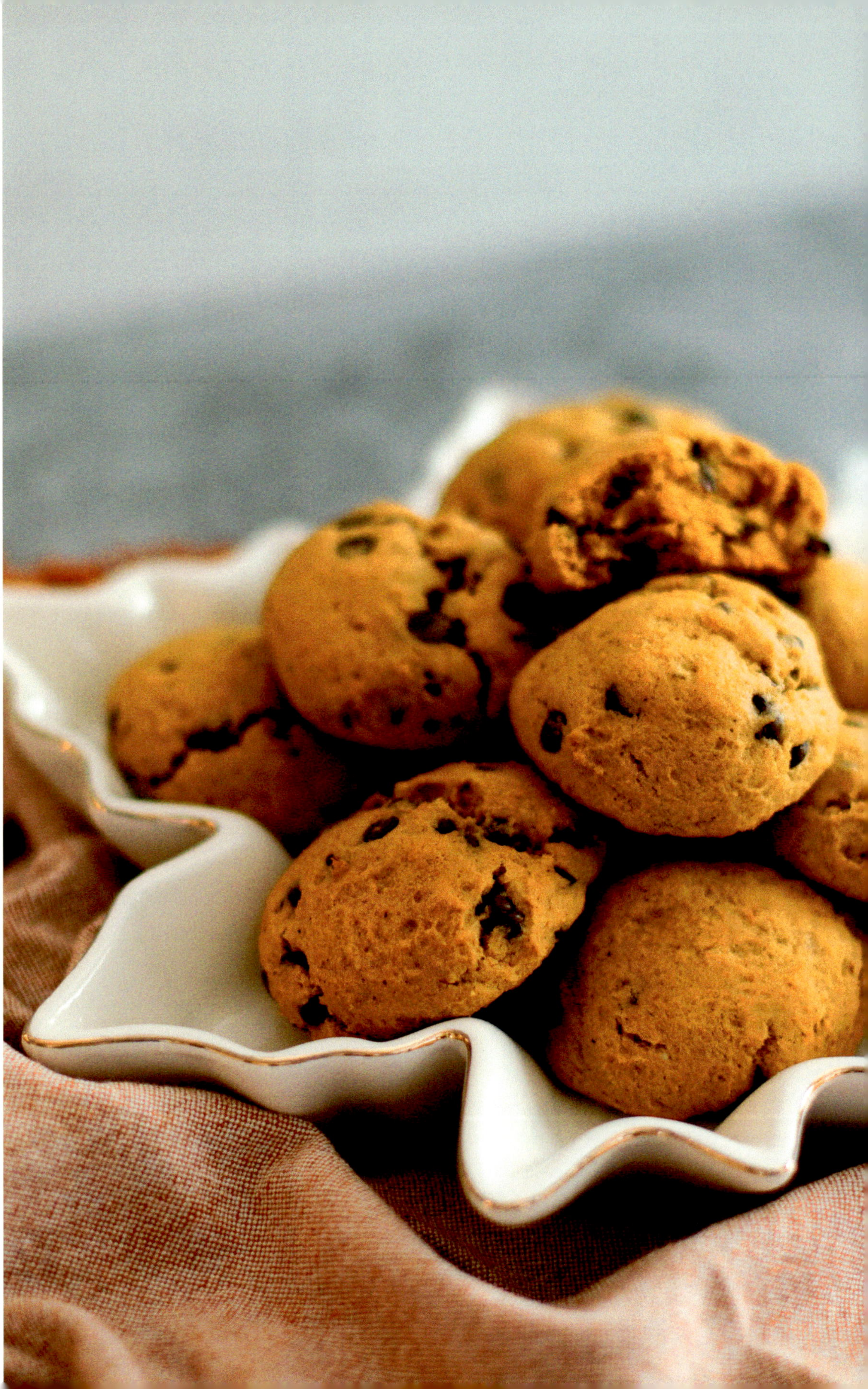

Egg Free

Nut Free

Gluten Free

Soy Free

GF Pumpkin Chocolate Chip Cookies

A soul-warming cup of coffee, a crisp chill in the air, the season outside is changing, and these cookies were made for the fall baking season. I've discovered keeping them in the fridge and eating them chilled reminds me of eating cookie dough even when I know I shouldn't. Together with the slight crunch of the mini chocolate chips, the soft texture gives these cookies the perfect excuse to enjoy anytime during the fall season. The best part? Gluten, egg, nut, and soy-free, these cookies don't need to be eaten in secrecy like raw cookie dough.

OVERALL PREP TIME: 25-30 minutes

CHILL TIME: 15-20 minutes

COOK TIME: 16-19 minutes

YIELDS: 14 cookies

Ingredients:

½ cup butter, softened

½ cup packed light brown sugar

½ cup canned pumpkin puree

1 tsp pure vanilla extract

1 cup 1:1 gluten-free flour

2 tsp pumpkin pie spice

1 tsp baking powder

Pinch of salt

½ cup semi-sweet mini chocolate chips

Directions:

- Preheat the oven to 350 degrees Fahrenheit. Prepare a baking sheet with parchment paper.
- In a large mixing bowl, using an electric mixer, cream together the butter and sugar until light and fluffy. Add the pumpkin puree and vanilla and continue to beat together until thick and well incorporated (1-2 minutes).
- In a separate bowl, whisk together the gluten-free flour, pumpkin pie spice, baking powder, and salt.
- While using the electric mixer, slowly incorporate the dry ingredients into the pumpkin mixture. Finally, fold in the chocolate chips.
- Chill dough in the refrigerator for at least 15-20 minutes.
- After the dough is chilled, begin rolling into individual dough balls (1 - 1 ½ inches) and place on the prepared baking sheet.
- Bake 16-19 minutes and let cool before serving.

Tips:

Store in an airtight container in the refrigerator for up to 5-6 days
Can be made with regular all-purpose flour in place of gluten-free flour; use 1:1 ratio.

☆☆☆☆☆

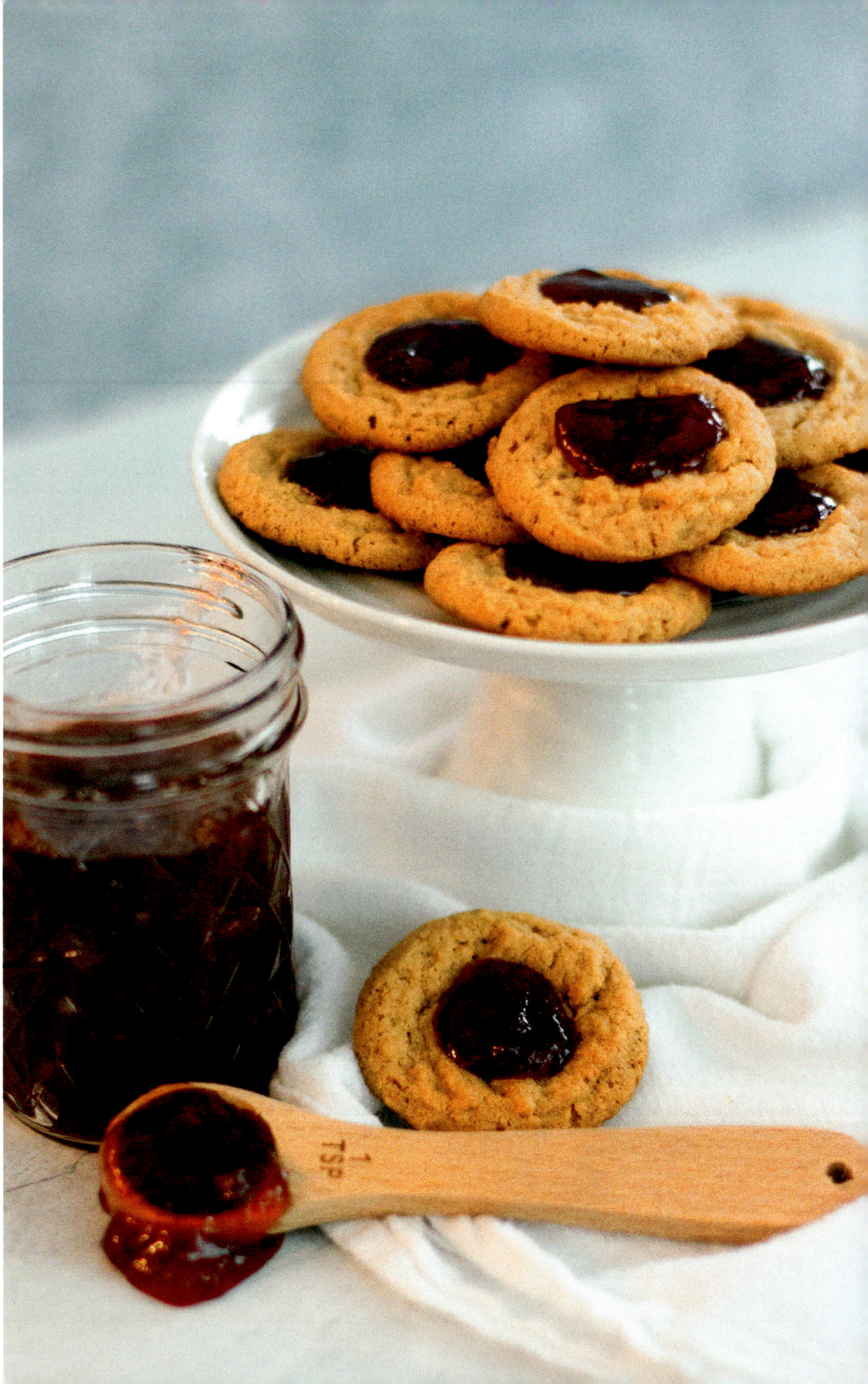

Egg Free

Gluten Free

Soy Free

GF Emmie's Mini PB&J Cookies

Looking for a kid's cookie that is healthy enough to let them have two? You've landed on the right page, my friend. My Emmie girl LOVES a stuffed almond butter and jelly sandwich any day of the week so I knew her palette would enjoy these simple yet delicious cookies as well. Little did I know just how much she would enjoy them.. When I let her try the first batch, she gobbled it up like a goldfish gulps water. The best trick I have for making these kid-friendly is the size. I use an extra-small ice cream scoop (#100 or 2 tsp), allowing Emmie to enjoy a sweet treat without giving her an overload of sugar. In addition, these cookies are gluten-free, egg-free, and soy-free, which provides more freedom if you're planning on bringing cookies to share at school or other functions where there are known allergies.

OVERALL PREP TIME: 40 minutes

INACTIVE PREP TIME: 25 minutes to chill dough

COOK TIME: 11-12 minutes

YIELDS: 60+ cookies

Ingredients:

½ cup butter, softened

1 cup creamy style almond butter *(or peanut butter)*

1 cup packed light brown sugar

¼ cup unsweetened applesauce

1 tsp pure vanilla extract

1 cup 1:1 gluten free flour

1 tsp baking soda

1 tsp baking powder

Pinch of salt

Jelly/jam of choice for the center *(grape, strawberry, etc)*

Directions:

- In a large mixing bowl, add the softened butter and almond butter. Using a spatula, mix together until smooth and creamy. Add the brown sugar, apple sauce, and vanilla and continue to mix until well combined.
- In a separate mixing bowl, combine the flour, baking soda, baking powder, and pinch of salt.
- Combine the flour mixture to the wet ingredients and mix until well combined.
- Chill the dough in the refrigerator for at least 25 minutes. Can be chilled overnight if you're making these ahead of time.
- While the dough is chilling, preheat the oven to 350 degrees Farenheit and prepare 2 baking sheets with parchment paper.
- Using an extra-small ice cream scoop (2tsp or #100), begin scooping dough onto a prepared baking sheet. Dough will not spread too much, so feel free to pack the cookies closer together.
- Bake for 11-12 minutes or until lightly golden brown and slight cracks begin to appear.
- Take the cookies out of the oven. Using the back of a teaspoon, gently press an indention into the middle of the cookie. While still warm, place a small dollop of preferred jelly in the center.
- Let cool completely before transferring to a plate or serving.

Tip:

Store in the refrigerator for up to one week

☆☆☆☆☆

STEPH'S family favorite TOP PICK

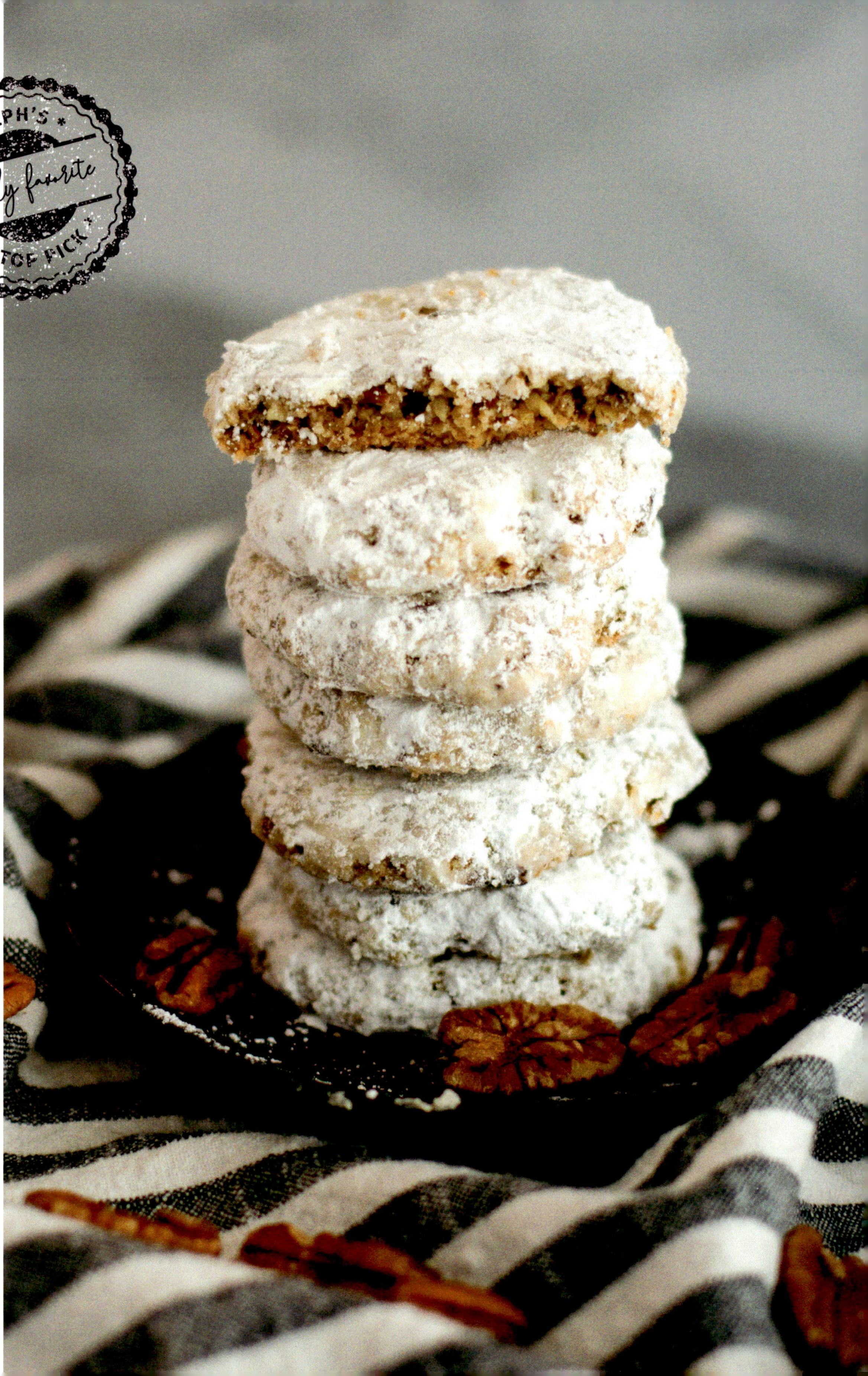

Egg Free

Gluten Free

Soy Free

GF Simple Pecan Sandies

Every Christmas season my mom makes her traditional "snowball" cookies, which essentially are Mexican wedding cookies. She doesn't have many cookies in her repertoire, but the ones she does bake up are top notch and worth being present to consume while still warm. It's become a tradition for our family, knowing that the kitchen will be smelling like snowball cookies come the month of December. She doesn't just make them for us, no, she makes more than enough to hand out to almost everybody she crosses paths with during the entire Christmas season. That's my mom, always giving and ALWAYS thinking of others.

After going gluten-free myself, I was on a mission to develop a similar recipe without the flour. With a few tries and several sweet taste testings later, these simple pecan sandies quickly became one of my favorites in this book. They are crunchy, crumbly, and melt in your mouth. The same kind of delicious that allows family traditions to still thrive even if you have dietary restrictions.

OVERALL PREP TIME: 20 minutes

INACTIVE PREP TIME: 20-30 mins to chill dough

COOK TIME: 20 minutes

YIELDS: 24 cookies

Ingredients:

¾ cup butter, softened

¾ cup granulated sugar

2 tsp pure vanilla extract

2 cups ground oatmeal flour
(using a food processor, measure out 3 cups of rolled oats to be ground)

1 ½ tsp baking powder

1 ¾ cups finely chopped pecans
(using a food processor, measure out 2 cups of pecans)

2 cups confectioners' sugar for dusting on top

Tip:

Store in an airtight container for up to 6 days.

Directions:

PREP: Grind rolled oats into flour and chop pecans into fine pieces - using food processor.

- Preheat the oven to 325 degrees Farenheit and prepare a baking sheet with parchment paper.
- Cream together the butter and sugar until light and fluffy. Add the vanilla and continue to beat until incorporated.
- In a separate bowl, combine the oatmeal flour, baking powder, and chopped pecans. Whisk until incorporated.
- Slowly add the oat flour mixture to the butter mixture (½ at a time) and mix until just combined and no dry flour is visible.
- Chill in the fridge for at least 20-30 minutes. Can be chilled overnight to be used the next day as well.
- Once the dough is chilled, begin rolling dough into 1" balls and place on the prepared baking sheet. Using your palm, lightly flatten the balls before baking.
- Bake for 20-22 minutes
- While the cookies are baking, sift the confectioners' sugar into a small bowl.
- After the cookies have baked and are still warm (warm enough to hold without falling apart). Place on a cooling rack to continue to cool.

*If desired, roll the cookies in the confectioners' sugar a second time to thoroughly coat.

☆☆☆☆☆

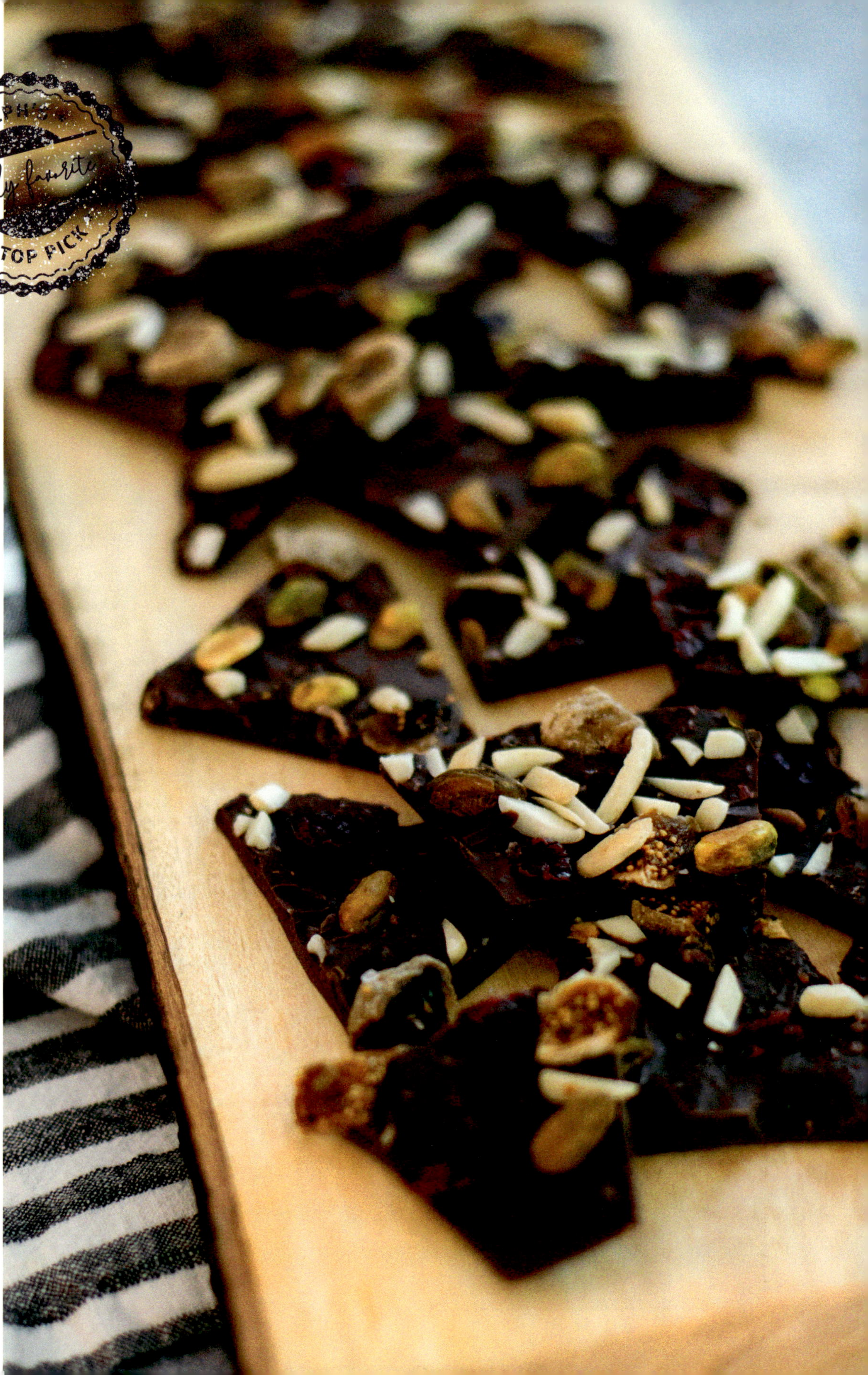

STEPH'S family favorite TOP PICK

Dairy Free

Gluten Free

Egg Free

Soy Free

GF Steph's Antioxidant Chocolate Bark

Craving something sweet but still want to get those health benefits? Usually the two domains do not coincide very nicely, and it leaves us choosing one or the other. However, my mantra in life is constantly seeking the balance between taste and nutrition, yes, even with dessert. This chocolate bark uses semi-sweet chocolate, which still retains quite a bit of cocoa. Cocoa is high in flavonol (antioxidant) content. This property alone can help boost our antioxidant system, reduce inflammation, blood pressure, and LDL cholesterol. In addition, I've added cranberries (rich in fiber and flavonoids that help fight bacteria), figs (rich in fiber, magnesium, manganese, calcium, iron, and anti-inflammatory compounds), pistachios (rich in copper, manganese, vitamin B6, fiber, phosphorus, thiamine and carotenoids), and almonds (rich in monounsaturated healthy fats and help promote healthy digestive tract & immune function). All together with a hint of pink himalayan salt, these chocolate bark bites will have you reaching for more without feeling any guilt. I can honestly say these were my favorite sweet-treat during pregnancy and I hope you enjoy them just as much as I do.

PREP TIME: 15 minutes

CHILL TIME: 1+ hour

COOK TIME: No bake

YIELDS: 20-30 pieces

Ingredients:

1 (10oz) bag of semisweet chocolate chips

2 tsp liquid coconut oil

½ tsp pure vanilla extract

3 tsp granulated sugar

¼ cup dried cranberries

⅓ cup dried finely chopped figs

¼ cup shelled pistachios

¼ cup sliced almonds

1-2 tsp coarse/flaky pink himalayan salt

Directions:

- Prepare a large baking sheet with parchment paper, set aside for later.
- In a microwave safe bowl, empty the bag of chocolate chips. Melt the chips in the microwave for 2 minutes, stirring after each minute with a spatula.
- Add the coconut oil, vanilla extract, and sugar and stir to combine. Place back in the microwave and melt for another 30 seconds.
- Using the spatula, spread the melted chocolate smoothly over the parchment paper in a rectangular shape. It should be thin, but not a paper thin layer.
- In an even fashion, sprinkle the chopped dried fruit on top of the chocolate while still warm. Next, add the nuts. Lastly, sprinkle the salt.
- Using the back of a flat spatula, gently press the fruit/nuts into the chocolate. This allows for the pieces to submerge slightly without falling off once cooled.
- Place in the refrigerator to chill for at least 1 hour (longer is preferable). When the chocolate is set, simply use your hands to break the chocolate into as many pieces as desired.

Tips:

Store in the fridge for up to 10 days.
It can be stored in the freezer for later use as well.

☆☆☆☆☆

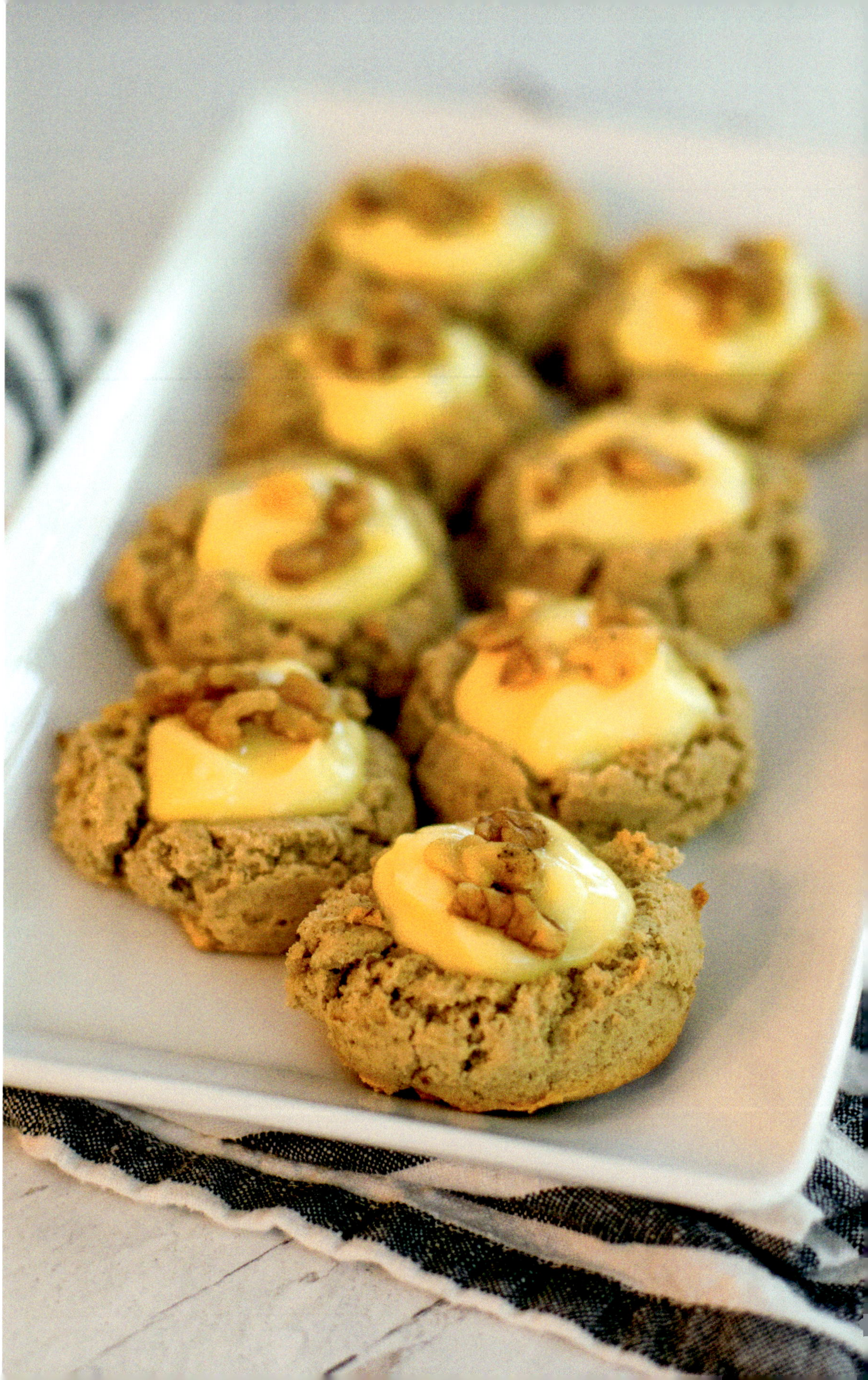

Gluten Free

Egg Free

Soy Free

GF Chunky Monkey Banana Pudding Cookies

Does your little one love bananas as much as mine does? She's gone through both phases of loving them and tossing them aside, but one thing that remains certain is the taste of familiarity. These days, she loves anything with bananas or banana flavor, from banana yogurt to banana popsicles; she's all in. I think most of us can agree, the taste of bananas is so familiar and universal. We either land on one side or the other -- loving them or tossing them. For those of you who love bananas and anything banana-flavored, these cookies are a must-make. They are especially fun for kids to make because the pudding mix is an easy way to get them involved without daunting instructions or a multitude of ingredients to clean up. If you want to make the cookies taste even more like a traditional banana pudding, add crushed vanilla wafers on top as a crowd-pleaser. Personally, I stuck with chopped walnuts to get some omega-3 fatty acid benefits.

PREP TIME: 20 minutes

INACTIVE PREP TIME: 1 hour to chill dough

COOK TIME: 10-11 minutes

YIELDS: 20 cookies

Ingredients:

½ cup butter, softened

½ cup granulated sugar

¾ cup mashed banana (about 1 ½ large bananas)

1 tsp pure vanilla extract

2 cups 1:1 gluten free flour (or regular all purpose flour)

1 tsp baking powder

1 tsp baking soda

1 tsp ground cinnamon

Pinch of coarse kosher salt

1 (3.4 oz) Jell-O™ Banana Cream Flavor Instant Pudding Mix

2 cups milk

Optional: Chopped walnuts or crushed vanilla wafers for topping

☆☆☆☆☆

Directions:

- In a large mixing bowl, using an electric mixer, cream together the butter and sugar until light and fluffy (about 1-2 minutes). Add the mashed banana and continue to mix on medium speed until consistency is somewhat smooth and even. Add the vanilla and mix until just combined.
- In a separate small mixing bowl, combine the GF flour, baking soda, baking powder, cinnamon, and pinch of salt.
- Combine the flour mixture to the wet ingredients and mix until well combined.
- Using a Scoop #40 (1 ½ inches size), begin scooping out cookie balls onto a large baking sheet. (You will chill the dough before baking so there is no need to space the cookies out yet.)
- Once the dough is scooped out into pre-measured balls, place the baking sheet in the refrigerator for 1 hour to chill. This allows the butter to set and prevent the cookies from spreading too much.
- While the cookies are chilling, prepare the banana pudding according to directions on the package: Whisk together the instant pudding powder with 2 cups milk until slightly thickened. Place in the refrigerator for the remainder of time the cookies are chilling/ baking.
- Once the cookie dough is chilled, preheat the oven to 350 degrees Fahrenheit and prepare another baking sheet with parchment paper. Transfer about 10-12 cookies to the prepared baking sheet and bake for 10-11 minutes or until slightly golden brown.
- While the cookies are still hot, using the back of a tablespoon, gently press into the cookies to create a "concave" or bowl shape. You may need to slightly reshape the edges of the cookies with your fingers.
- Place a dollop of chilled banana pudding in the center of each cookie and top with optional chopped walnuts or crushed vanilla wafers.
- Repeat with the second batch of cookies.

Tips:

Best served chilled.
Store in the refrigerator for up to 7 days.

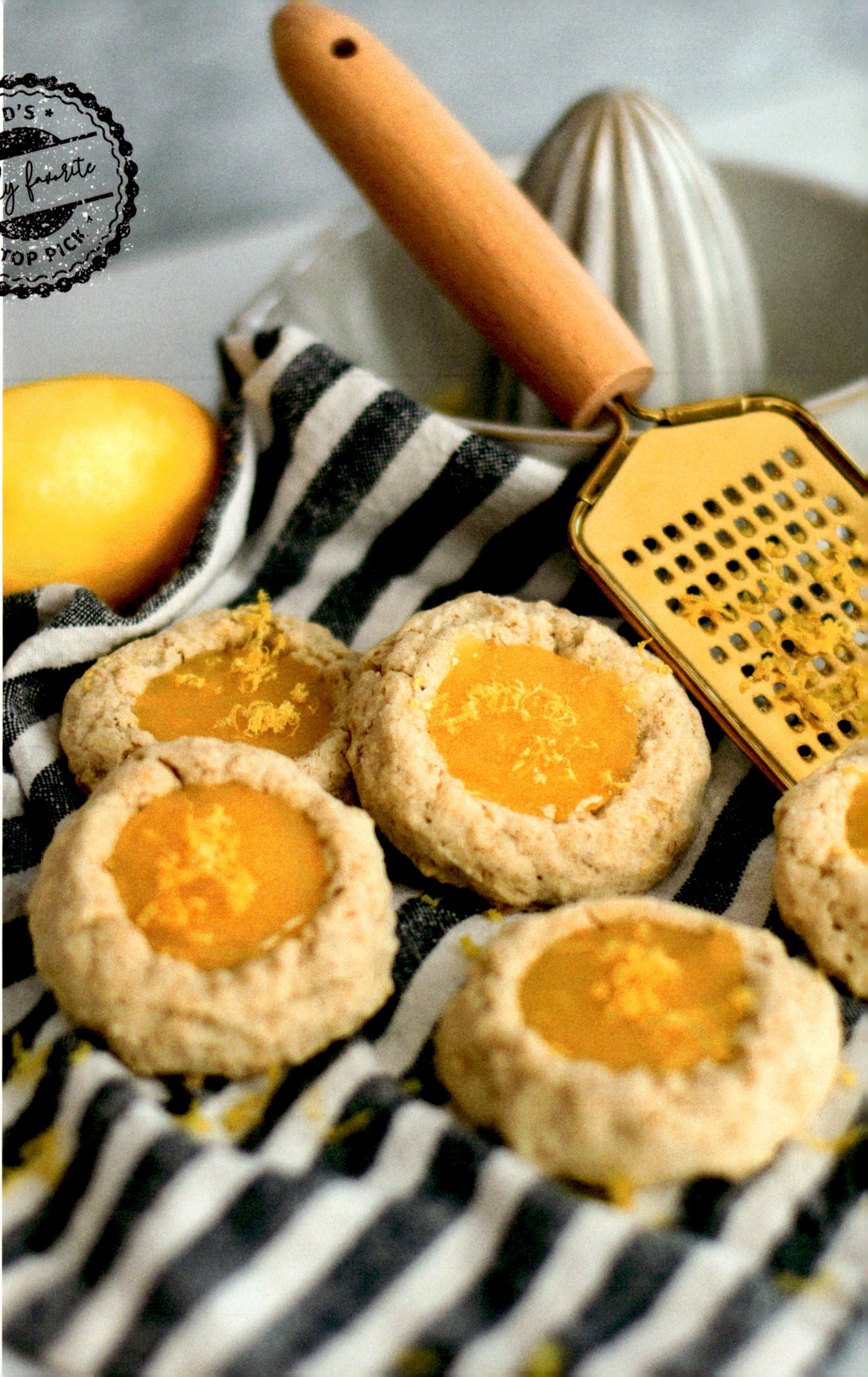

Nut Free

Gluten Free

Soy Free

GF Fresh Lemon Curd Cookies

I'm not sure there is anything more refreshing than freshly squeezed lemon juice. I've always been a fan of lemon cookies, scones, muffins, cakes, you name it! One of my reasons for making these lemon curd cookies is wanting to create a cookie that that mimicked a lemon bar. You know, the ooey gooey lemon filling you can sink your teeth into? My first trial and major error ended in a cookie looking more like a dismal fried egg with a faint lemon flavor. I remember Justin and I looking at each other when I handed him a cookie for a taste test, he simply said, "This ain't it," without even taking a bite. I just laughed because I knew it was true. Since that cookie error, I've discovered that making the curd on the stove is key. Consistently whisking over medium heat and letting the curd really thicken up allows you to enjoy that same lemon bar experience I was originally going for.

PREP TIME: 20 minutes

COOK TIME: 15 minutes

YIELDS: 18 cookies

Ingredients:

COOKIE DOUGH

½ cup butter, softened

1 cup granulated sugar

1 large egg

1 tsp pure vanilla extract

1 ¼ cup 1:1 gluten-free flour

¾ cup quick oats

½ tsp salt

1 tsp baking powder

2 tbsp lemon zest

LEMON CURD FILLING

1 cup granulated sugar

2 large eggs

1 heaping tbsp lemon zest

3 tbsp fresh lemon juice

2 tbsp butter

Tip:

Store in the fridge for up to 1 week.

Directions:

PREP: Zest and juice 2-3 lemons .

*It's best to have all ingredients ready to go when baking the cookies and making the lemon curd. Lemon curd requires consistent whisking at the stove to prevent lumps.

- Preheat the oven to 325 degrees Fahrenheit and prepare a baking sheet with parchment paper.
- Cream together the butter and sugar until light and fluffy. Add the egg and vanilla and continue to beat until incorporated.
- In a separate bowl, whisk together the gluten-free flour, quick oats, salt, baking powder, and lemon zest.
- Slowly add the flour mixture to the butter mixture and mix until just combined and no dry flour is visible.
- Using a Scoop #40, scoop out the dough and place it on the prepared baking sheet—Bake for 15 minutes.
- While the cookies are baking, begin making the lemon curd on the stove.
- Heat a small saucepan over medium-high heat. Add the sugar and eggs and whisk together until combined. After 5-7 minutes of whisking the eggs, add the lemon juice and zest, continue to whisk to prevent lumps or burning. Once the curd has thickened slightly, turn the heat down to medium-low. Add the butter and continue to whisk until combined. Turn the heat off once the curd is at the desired thickness (it will take the same length of time as cookies are baking).
- After the cookies are done baking, press down in the center of the cookie while still warm to create a 'bowl' shape using the back of a tbsp.
- Scoop out lemon curd and pour into the center of the cookie.

*Garnish with additional lemon zest if desired.

☆☆☆☆☆

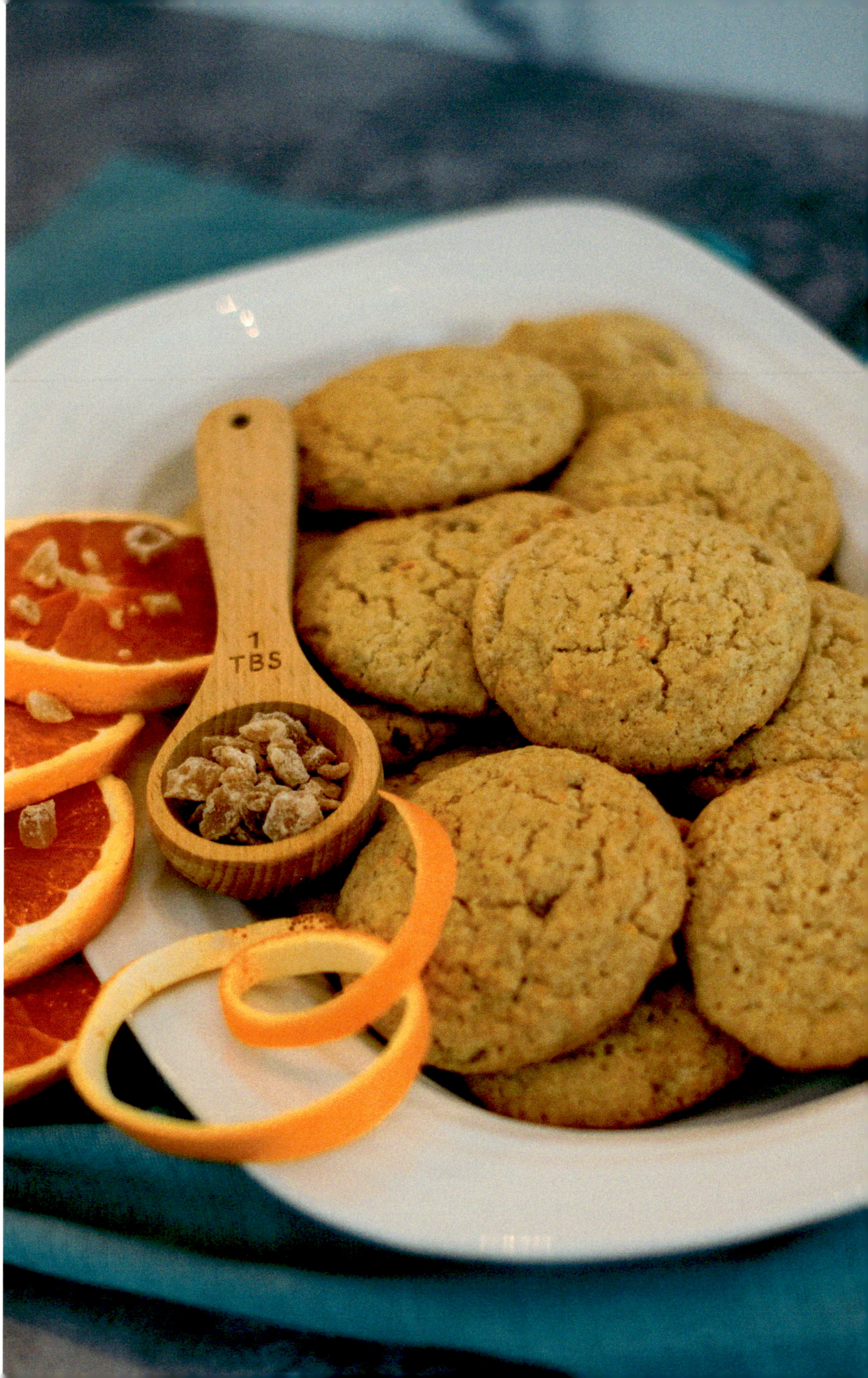

Egg Free

Gluten Free

Soy Free

GF Candied Orange Ginger Cookies

Going through pregnancy has it's fair share of symptoms, one overall theme being nausea at some point or another. For me, I always got nauseated in the afternoons. Ginger, however, has been used for centuries to alleviate nausea and stomach upset (whether pregnant or not). In addition, ginger contains phytonutrients such as antioxidants and anti-inflammatories that make this ingredient worth investing in and adding to your favorite dishes and even desserts. These cookies are among my favorites because the candied ginger is a subtle flavor in the background that complements the sweet taste of fresh orange. If you can't find candied or crystallized ginger in the stores, try using ground ginger instead.

PREP TIME: 15 minutes

COOK TIME: 15 minutes

YIELDS: 24 cookies

Ingredients:

½ cup butter, softened

1 cup granulated sugar

½ cup unsweetened applesauce

1 tsp pure vanilla extract

¼ cup freshly squeezed orange juice

1 ½ cup 1:1 gluten free flour

¾ cup almond flour

½ tsp baking powder

½ tsp baking soda

Pinch of salt

Zest of 1 large orange (about 1 ½ tbsp)

⅓ cup crystalized or candied ginger

Directions:

- Preheat the oven to 350 degrees Fahrenheit and prepare a baking sheet with parchment paper.
- Cream together the butter and sugar until light and fluffy. Add the applesauce and vanilla and continue to beat until incorporated. Lastly, add the orange juice.
- In a separate bowl, combine the gluten free flour, almond flour, baking powder, baking soda, salt, and orange zest. Whisk until incorporated.
- Slowly add the flour mixture to the butter mixture (half at a time) and mix until just combined and no dry flour is visible.
- Fold in the candied ginger.
- Using a Scoop #100, begin scooping dough into 1" balls and place on the prepared baking sheet. Dough will be slightly sticky and hard to ball up without an ice cream scoop.
- Bake for 15 minutes

Tips:

Can store in the fridge or on the countertop for 5-6 days.

If placed in an airtight container on the countertop, the cookies will become softer over time.

☆☆☆☆☆

Egg Free

Nut Free

Dairy Free

Gluten Free

Soy Free

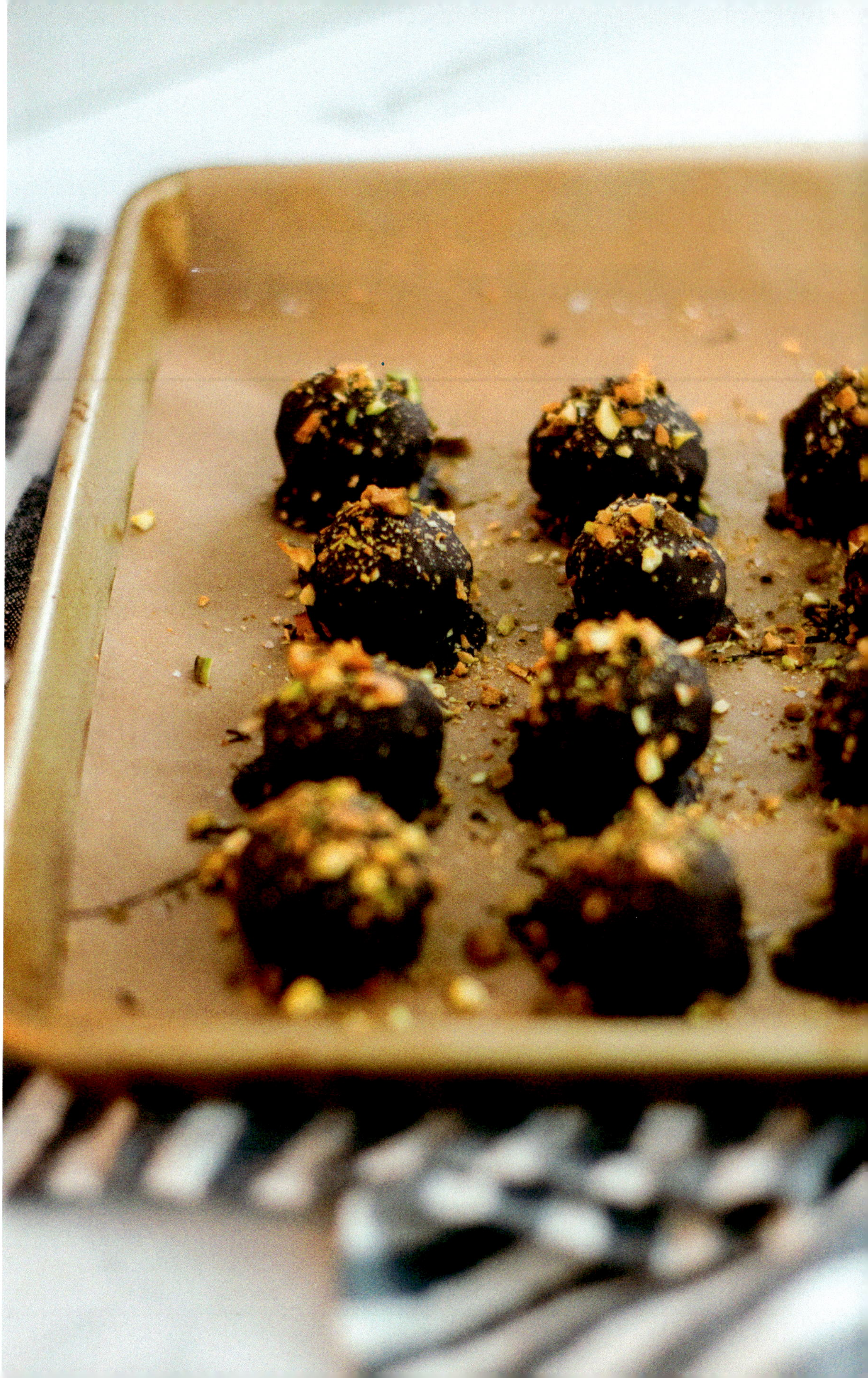

GF No Bake Figgy Pops

If your lifestyle calls for simplicity with desserts and needing options with no added sugars, I highly recommend these no-bake cookies. They are simply delicious and packed full of nutrients with the figs, dates, almond butter, and pistachios. These are some of the easiest cookies to make in this book but that doesn't mean the taste is ordinary. Throughout my pregnancy, I enjoyed these plenty of times as a mid-day snack to suppress the need for something sweet yet not too decadent that would send my blood sugar into overdrive. In addition, the fiber content from the figs, dates, and pistachios make these cookies a great option for diabetics or anybody else watching their added sugar intake.

PREP TIME: 20 minutes

COOK TIME: No bake

CHILL TIME: 1+ hour

YIELDS: 15 balls

Ingredients:

1 cup dried figs, stemmed and coarsely chopped

1 cup dried dates, stemmed and coarsely chopped

2 tbsp creamy style almond butter (or peanut butter)

1 cup semi-sweet chocolate chips

2 tsp coconut oil

2 tsp finely chopped pistachios

Dash flaky pink Himalayan salt

Directions:

- Prepare a small baking sheet with parchment paper.
- Using a food processor, add the chopped figs, dates, and almond butter. Pulse together until a moist, crumbly texture is formed (about 2-3 minutes).
- Using a tablespoon, scoop out the cookie dough mixture and shape into small balls. Place them on the prepared baking sheet.
- In a microwavable glass bowl, melt the chocolate chips and coconut oil for about 1 minute in the microwave. Using a spatula, mix well until all the lumps are gone.
- Using 2 forks, gently roll the shaped cookie balls into the chocolate and place them back on the prepared baking sheet.
- Sprinkle the tops with the chopped pistachios and flaky Himalayan salt before they dry.
- Place the baking sheet in the fridge to set for at least 1 hour.

Tips:

Best served chilled.
Store in the fridge for up to 10 days.
It can be stored in the freezer for later use as well.

☆☆☆☆☆

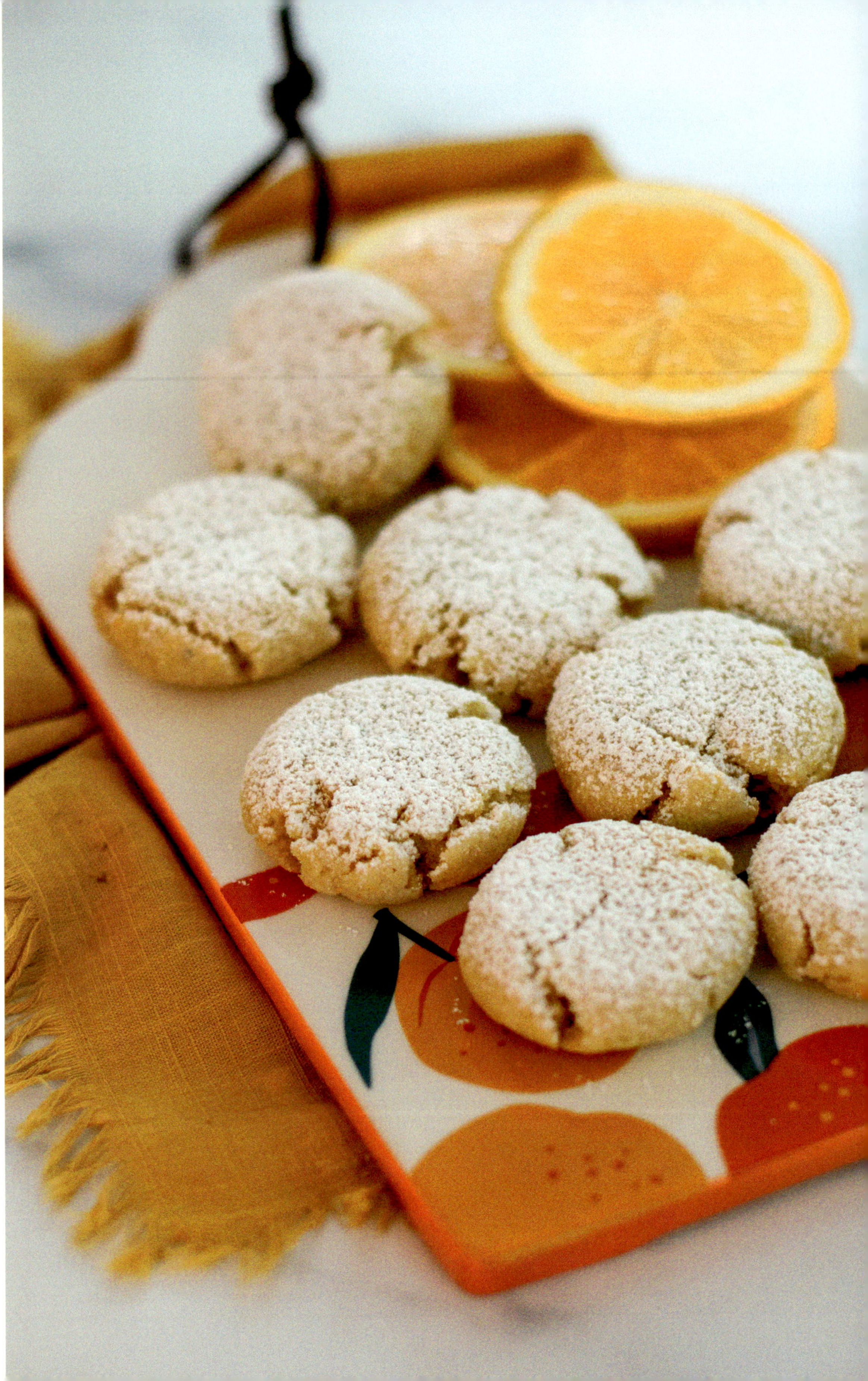

Dairy Free

Gluten Free

Soy Free

GF Chewy Orange Almond Cookies

One of my first cookie recipes that dates back several years ago is these orange almond cookies that are incredibly simple to make. The simplicity of ingredients has you coming back for more with no guilt or strings attached. I love that these cookies don't require an electric mixer to make or contain dairy products. One of my only recipes that don't contain dairy, these cookies make a great option for anybody with allergies. They taste so light and fresh--better gobble them before somebody else smells fresh orange cookies baking in the kitchen.

PREP TIME: 20 minutes

COOK TIME: 17-18 minutes

YIELDS: 14-15 cookies

Ingredients:

2 cups almond flour

½ cup granulated sugar

1 large orange, zested

2 large egg whites

½ tsp cream of tartar

1 tsp pure vanilla extract

½ tsp pure almond extract

Optional topping:
Confectioner's sugar

Directions:

- Preheat the oven to 325 degrees Fahrenheit and prepare a baking sheet with parchment paper.
- In a medium-sized mixing bowl, whisk together the almond flour, sugar, and orange zest.
- In a separate bowl, combine the egg whites, cream of tartar, vanilla extract, and almond extract. Whisk quickly and thoroughly until foamy and soft peaks form (about 5-8 minutes of quick whisking).
- Pour the wet ingredients into the flour mixture and fold them together using a rubber spatula until well-combined.
- Roll into 1" balls and place on the prepared baking sheet. These cookies will not spread; you can place them closer together to save room.
- Bake for 15 minutes. While still in the oven, take a metal spatula and gently smash them down until about ½" thick. Continue to bake for another 2-3 minutes.
- Let cookies cool completely before topping with confectioner's sugar. If using the confectioner's sugar, use a small sieve to sprinkle a light dusting of sugar over the tops of the cookies.

Tips:

Serve at room temperature.
Store in the refrigerator for 5-6 days.

☆☆☆☆☆

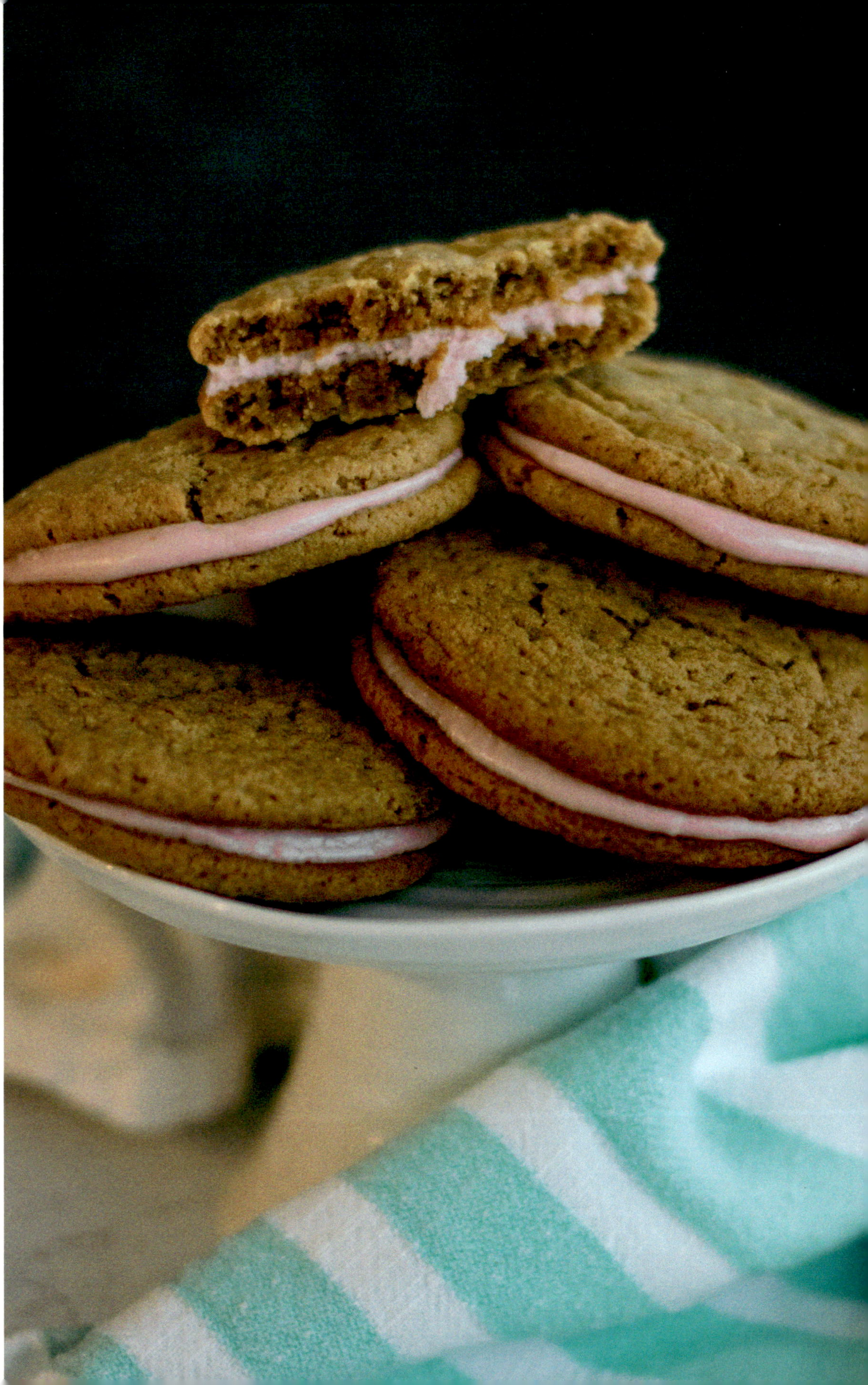

Egg Free

Gluten Free

Soy Free

Nutty n' Pink Whoopies (Baby Shower / Baby Reveal cookies)

These cookies were a cookie accident when they first came out of the oven. I'll tell you, this was the beginning of my PB and J cookie recipe. Initially I was on the fence of throwing them out but then I had an idea that turned out to be one of my most delicious ones yet. These have since become one of my favorite cookies.
Have you ever had an oatmeal creme pie cookie? Of course you have, but have you had an almond butter creme pie cookie that negates including gluten, egg, and soy? Didn't think so! These take the traditional oatmeal creme pie cookies to the next level. Creating a flavor profile that is slightly salty but so incredibly sweet you can't stop yourself from eating the whole thing. The pink frosting color comes from grape jelly, but the taste is negligible and can't be detected. These make for perfect gender reveal and baby shower cookies, allowing you to change the frosting color without adding artificial colors or additives to your food. Don't want any color? Keep the jelly out of the frosting and you'll have a traditional creme pie cookie.

OVERALL PREP TIME: 1 hour

INACTIVE PREP TIME: 25 minutes to chill dough

COOK TIME: 12-13 minutes

YIELDS: 10 sandwich cookies

Ingredients:

½ cup butter, softened

1 cup creamy style almond butter (or peanut butter)

1 cup packed light brown sugar

¼ cup unsweetened applesauce

1 tsp pure vanilla extract

1 cup 1:1 gluten free flour

1 tsp baking soda

Pinch of salt

FILLING

2 cups confectioner's sugar

4 tbsp butter, softened

2 tbsp milk (unsweetened almond milk works well too)

3-4 tbsp grape jelly (depending on color/flavor preference)

☆☆☆☆☆

Directions:

- In a large mixing bowl, add the softened butter and almond butter. Using a spatula, mix together until smooth and creamy. Add the brown sugar, apple sauce, and vanilla and continue to mix until well combined.
- In a separate mixing bowl, combine the flour, baking soda, and pinch of salt.
- Combine the flour mixture to the wet ingredients and mix until well combined.
- Chill the dough in the refrigerator for at least 25 minutes. Can be chilled overnight if you're making these ahead of time.
- While the dough is chilling, preheat the oven to 350 degrees Fahrenheit and prepare a baking sheet with parchment paper.
- Roll into small ¾" - 1" balls and place on a baking sheet with room to spread.
- Bake for 12-13 minutes or until lightly golden brown and cracks begin to appear.
- Let cool completely before adding the filling.
- While the cookies are cooling begin making the filling. Using an electric mixer, whip together the confectioner's sugar and butter until semi-smooth consistency is formed. Add the milk and desired amount of grape jelly. You may have to stop the mixer several times to scoop down the edges of the bowl. I prefer to use 4 tbsp of jelly to create a bright pink frosting color. The taste of grape is negligible.
- After the cookies have cooled, simply spoon out the desired amount of filling and spread evenly on the bottom of one cookie. Using a second cookie, sandwich the filling together.

Tips:

Can be used for gender reveal parties, baby showers, etc.
To create a blue frosting color instead I suggest using blueberry jelly. This is a fun way to add coloring without using artificial colors and chemicals in your treats.
Can be served at room temperature or chilled. Store in the refrigerator for up to 1 week. Can be stored in the freezer for later use.

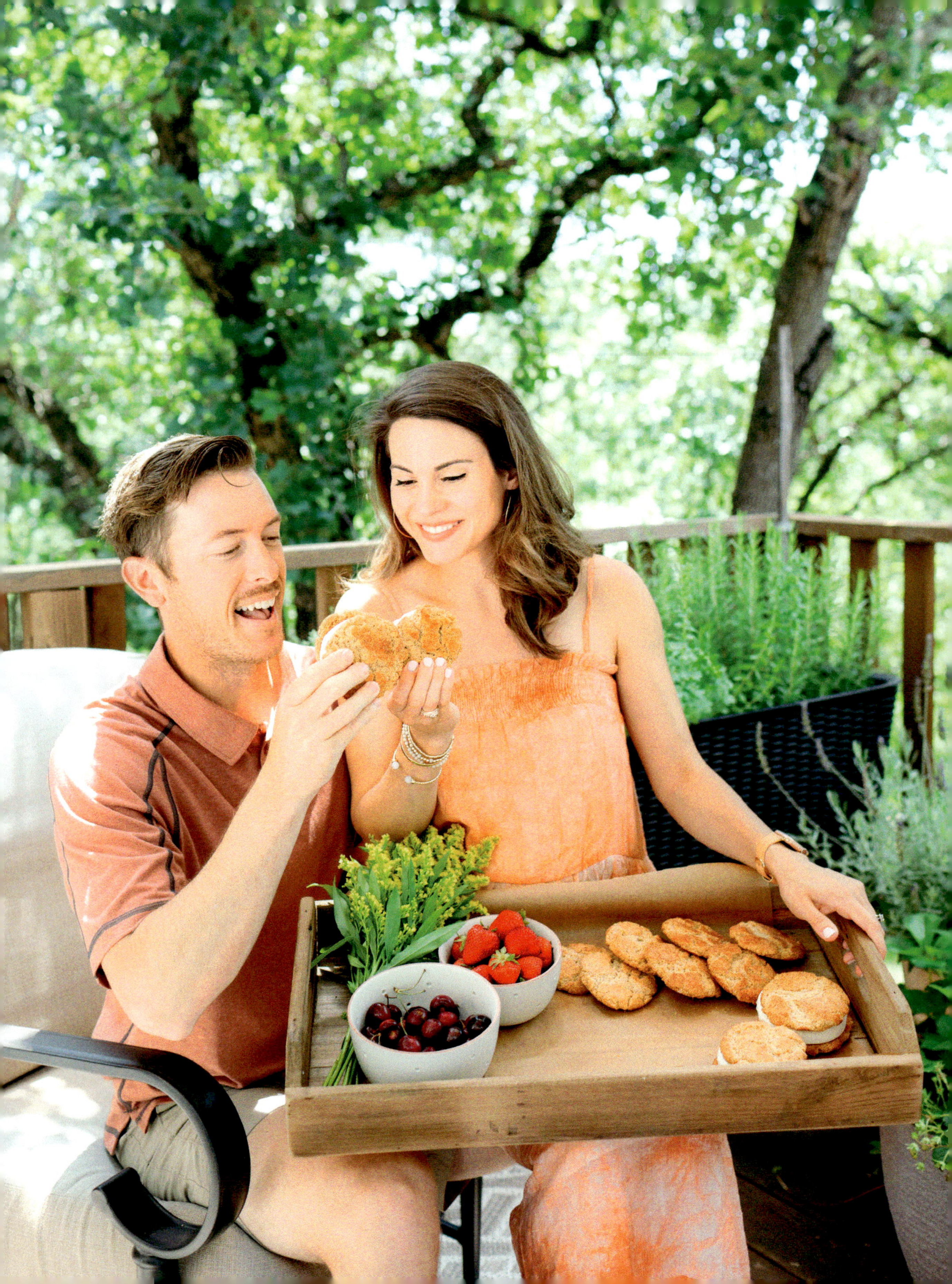

Cookies too Good to Pass up

- Drunk Rum Raisin Cookies
- Gooey Chewy S'mores Cookies
- Wake Me Up Espresso Chocolate Chip Cookies *(LFD's Pick)*
- Chocolate Thumbprint Cookies
- Dirty Bourbon Balls
- Chocolate Peanut Butter Smash Cookies
- Classic Snickerdoodle Ice Cream Sandwich Cookies
- Not So Traditional Oatmeal Chocolate Chip Cookies

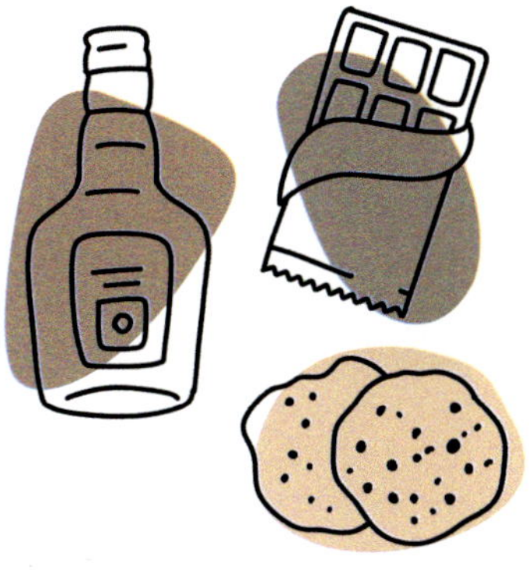

This section is all about the little indulgences in life. Yes, I am a firm believer in eating a variety of greens, drinking plenty of water, and getting substantial amounts of sleep; however, I still believe some desserts should be enjoyed without fussing too much about the ingredients. I can't say there's much nutritional value in these cookies, but I can say these cookies are simply valued as delicious.

After all, that is what makes a cookie, a cookie.

They've each been created with a different story and situation in mind, from adults only ingredients (rum & bourbon) to creating a kid's fantasy come true (S'mores & ice cream sandwiches). So the next time you're in the mood for a traditional, decadent cookie, these recipes will be your go-to choices.

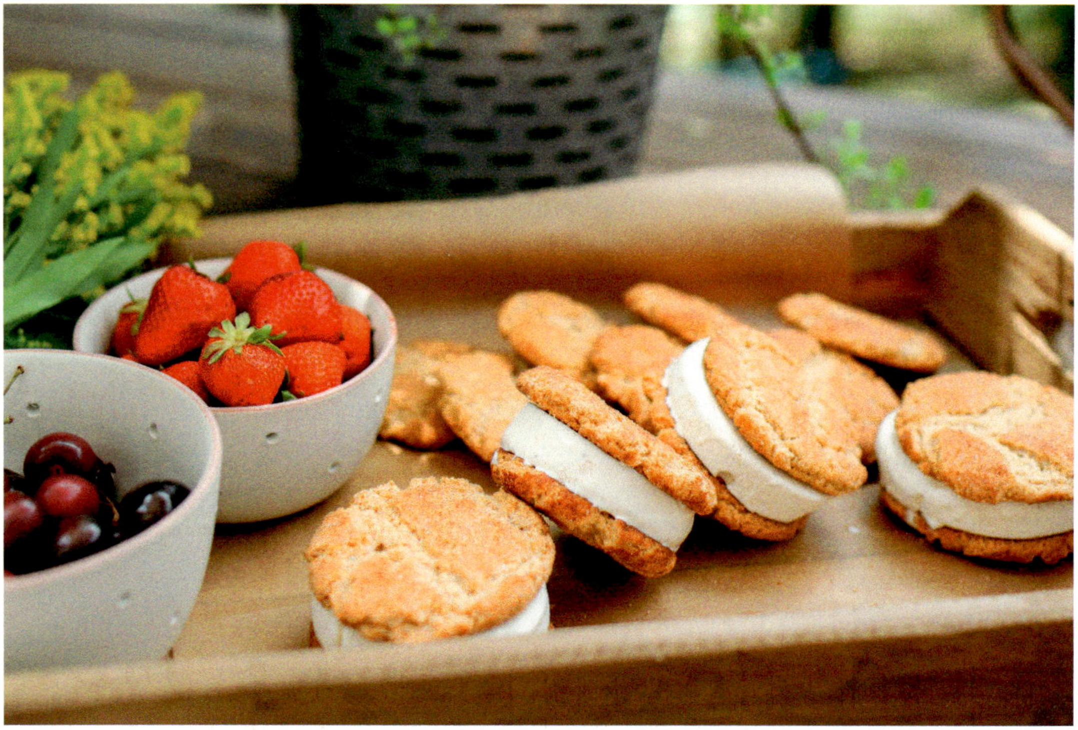

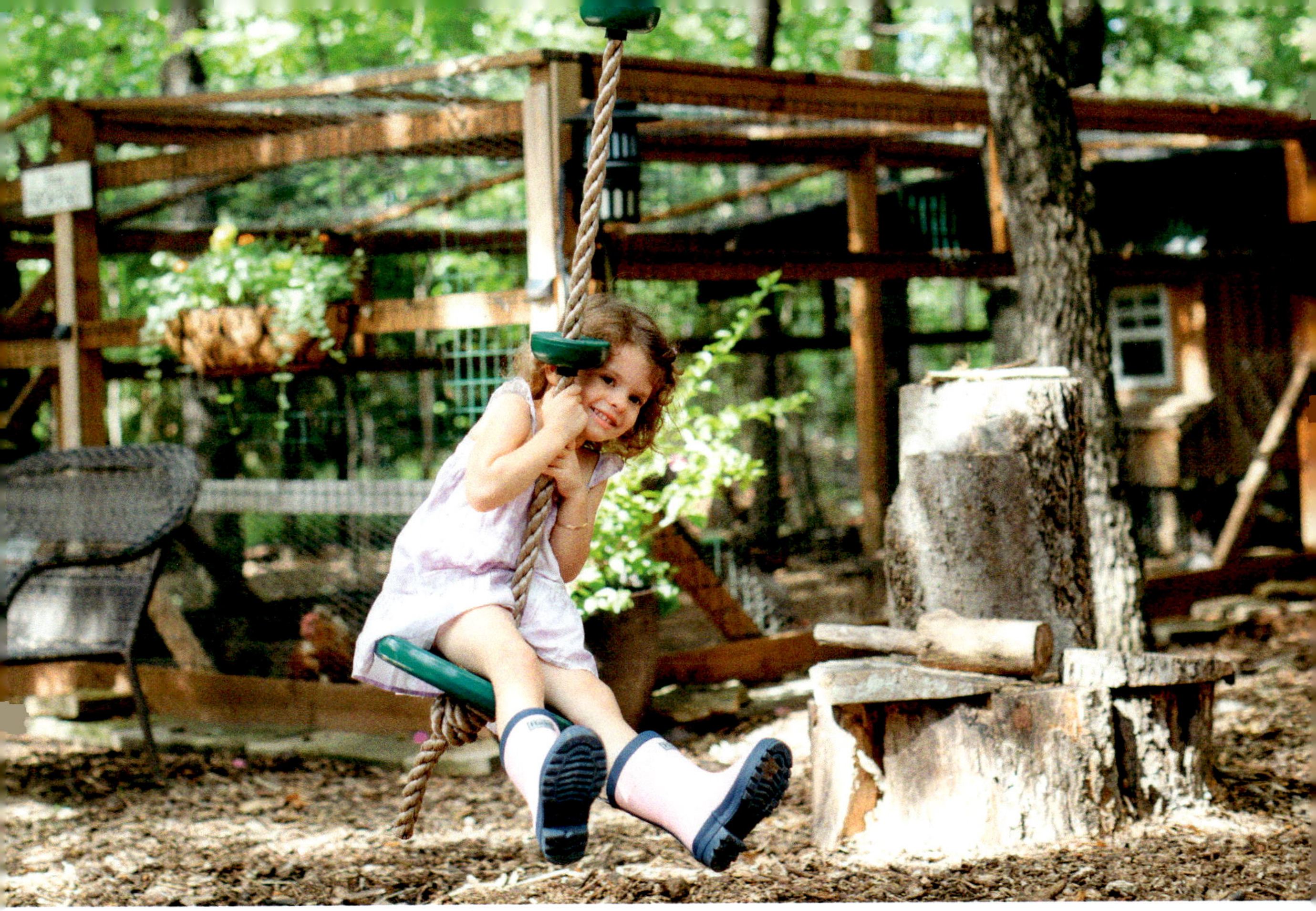

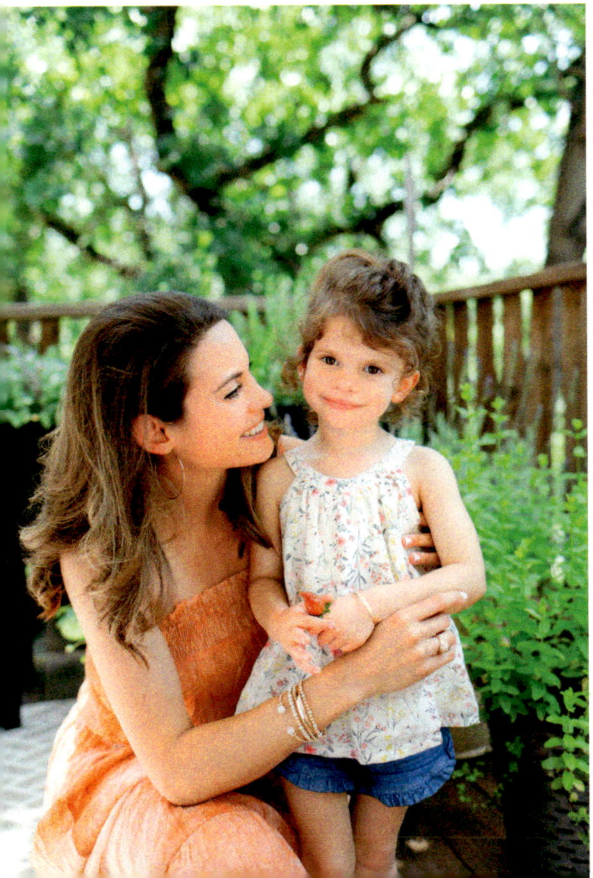

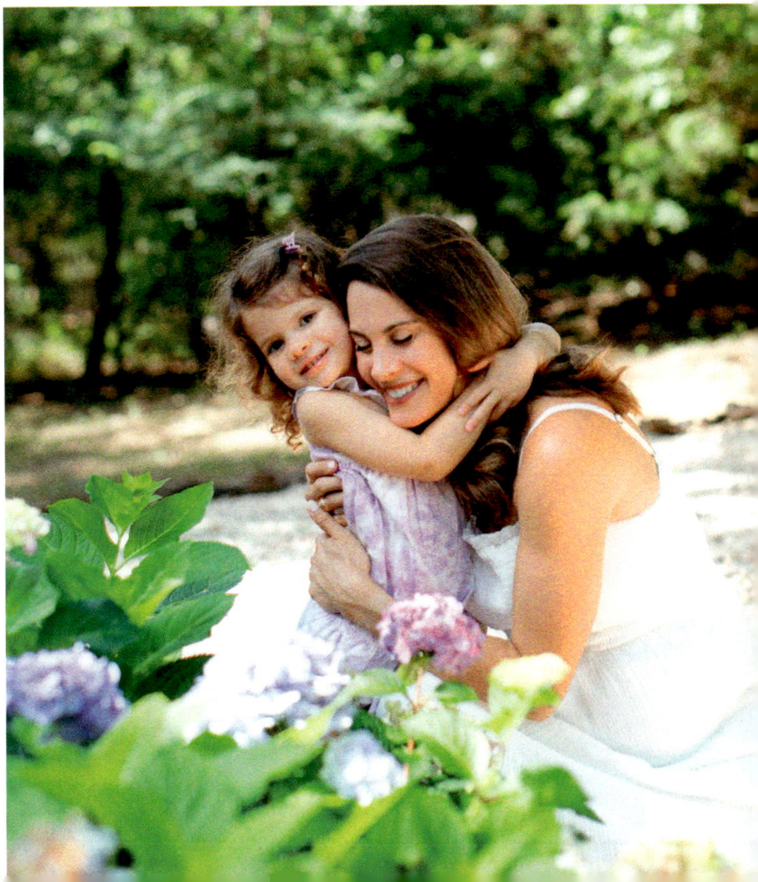

Drunk Rum Raisin Cookies

When I first began this cookie cookbook journey, I asked Justin what flavor he wanted to try the most. He confidently stated that a rum raisin cookie would be delightful and should make an appearance in this book. I agreed, although having never made a rum raisin cookie (or anything with that flavor, as a matter of fact), I went in search for some examples. Did y'all know there are a multitude of different ways to make rum raisin cookies? From rum raisin bread, to raisin pie, one thing is for certain: it all starts with a **dadgum good rum**! Our favorite rum brand is Bumbu™, hands down some of the best rum I've ever tasted. Imported from Barbados, this rum is crafted with sugarcane and spices from the West Indies, creating a unique yet traditional profile. It's smooth and flavorful, and hey having extra ingredients around to sample while whipping up these cookies might not be such a bad thing. After experimenting with my recipe several times, the fourth time was a charm. Not too much oatmeal, not too much flour, and just enough raisins and rum to leave you wanting more. Go ahead and take another; I won't tell a rummy secret.

PREP TIME: 20 minutes

INACTIVE PREP TIME: 1 hour to chill dough

COOK TIME: 12-13 minutes

YIELDS: 20 cookies

Ingredients:

¾ cup raisins

½ cup dark rum

½ cup butter, softened

1 cup packed light brown sugar

1 large egg

1 tsp pure vanilla extract

1 tsp rum extract

1 cup all purpose flour

1 cup old fashioned rolled oats

½ cup quick oats

1 tsp baking soda

2 tsp baking powder

Pinch of salt

Directions:

- Pour the raisins and rum in a small microwaveable bowl, making sure the raisins are submerged in the rum. Heat in the microwave for 1 minute and let cool.
- In a large mixing bowl, cream together the butter and brown sugar until light and fluffy (about 2 minutes). Add the egg, vanilla, and rum extracts and continue to mix until smooth.
- Add 2 tsp of the rum from the raisin bowl into the butter mixture.
- In a separate mixing bowl, combine the flour, oats, baking soda, baking powder, and pinch of salt.
- Combine the flour mixture with the wet ingredients and mix until just combined. Do not overmix, as this will cause your dough to be very sticky and mushy.
- Fold in the raisins.
- Place in the fridge to chill for about 1 hour OR in the freezer for about 20 minutes.
- While the dough is chilling, preheat the oven to 325 degrees Fahrenheit and prepare 2 cookie sheets with parchment paper.
- After the dough is chilled enough to handle (should be slightly chilled to the touch and less sticky), use a cookie scoop to drop cookies onto the prepared cookie sheets with room to spread.
- Bake for 12-13 minutes (depending on size) or until golden brown on the edges.

Tips:

Can be stored on the counter, uncovered.

If you choose to cover them in an airtight container, they will get softer and fall apart as time goes on.

Can be stored in the fridge as well.

☆☆☆☆☆

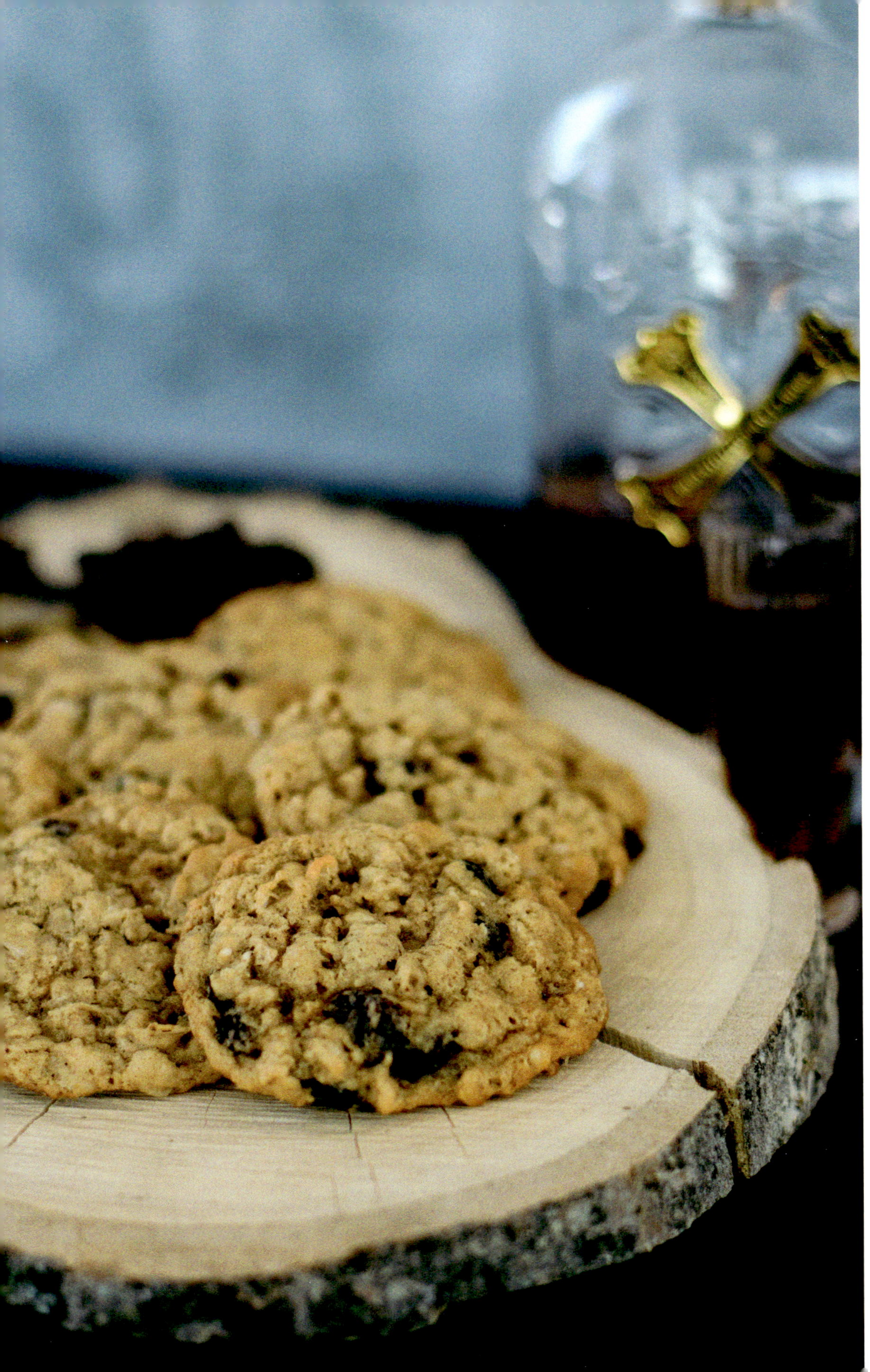

Nut Free

Soy Free

Gooey Chewy S'mores Cookies

I'll be honest, there's not much nutritional value in a s'mores treat, but the experience is what our inner child craves most. There's something about a traditional s'mores dessert that transports us back to a simpler time and age. For me, I grew up in Girl Scouts and no campout was ever complete without making a few DOZEN s'mores. The whole experience of roasting marshmallows over an open fire, learning how to rotate the stick so all edges get equally crystallized (but not burned), perfecting the pre-melted chocolate on the graham ahead of time. Whatever it is for you, s'mores can be very personal. This gives us each a memory we hold onto when we sink our teeth and taste buds into something similar. These cookies give you all of that plus the messy side, because what's a s'more without a marshmallow mess?

PREP TIME: 15 minutes

COOK TIME: 10-12 minutes

YIELDS: 21 cookies

Ingredients:

½ cup butter, softened

½ cup granulated sugar

½ packed light brown sugar

1 large egg

1 tsp pure vanilla extract

1 ¼ cup all purpose flour

1 tsp baking soda

1 tsp baking powder

Pinch of salt

1 cup mini marshmallows, plus additional for topping after baking

1 cup broken graham crackers

½ cup semi sweet chocolate chips

1 Hershey's™ bar broken into small pieces

Directions:

- Preheat the oven to 350 degrees Fahrenheit. Prepare 2 baking sheets with parchment paper.
- In a large mixing bowl, cream together the butter and both sugars until light and fluffy (about 1-2 minutes). Add the egg and vanilla and continue to beat until incorporated.
- In a separate mixing bowl, combine the flour, baking soda, baking powder, and pinch of salt.
- Combine the flour mixture to the wet ingredients and mix until well combined.
- Fold in the marshmallows, graham crackers, and chocolate chips.
- Using a 1" ice cream scoop, place cookies on a baking sheet with room to spread.
- Bake for 10 minutes, or until slightly underdone.
- Take the cookies out of the oven and place 2-3 more mini marshmallows and broken pieces of the Hershey's™ bar on top of the cookies. Place back in the oven for 1-2 minutes or until marshmallows are slightly melted and the chocolate is soft to give the desired s'more effect.

Tips:

Best served warm the day they are baked.

Store in an airtight container for up to 5 days.

☆☆☆☆☆

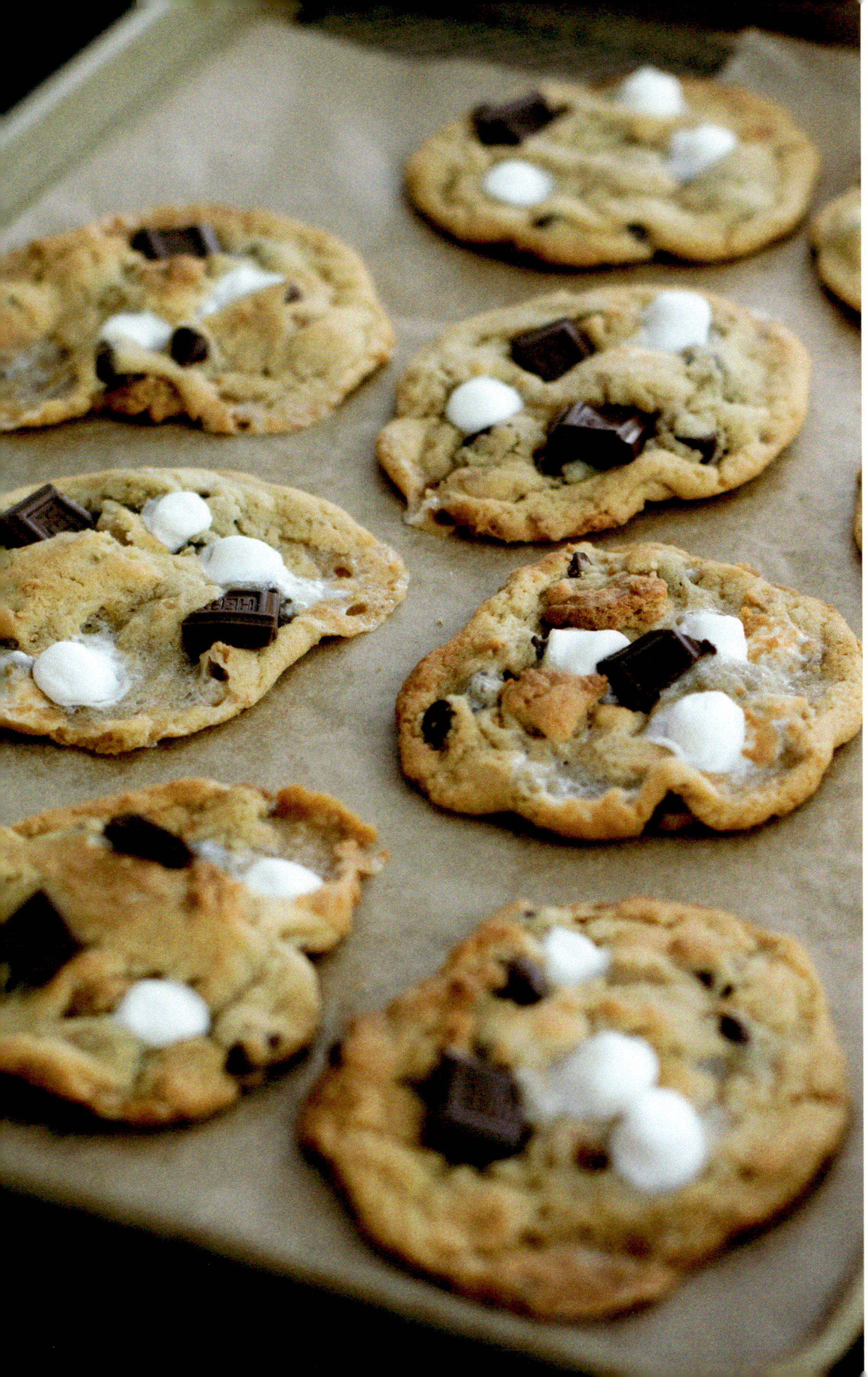

Wake Me Up Espresso Chocolate Chip Cookies

When we first invested in our espresso machine, my coffee drinking world suddenly opened up to endless opportunities. I am not a straight espresso shot drinker by any means, but I do occasionally enjoy a latte with a full espresso shot inside. Justin, on the other hand, can drink two dark roast espresso shots without a problem. These days, during my pregnancy, my coffee drinking has dwindled to nothing, but I still enjoy making these cookies with the smell of espresso lingering in the air. The cookie dough alone might make you think you're sitting in a coffee shop or perhaps a little bistro with fresh baked cookies & pastries.

PREP TIME: 15 minutes

INACTIVE PREP TIME: 1 hour to chill dough

COOK TIME: 13-15 minutes

YIELDS: 30 cookies

Ingredients:

1 cup butter, softened

1 cup packed light brown sugar

½ cup granulated sugar

1 large egg + 1 large egg yolk

4 tsp instant espresso powder

1 tsp pure vanilla extract

2 ½ cups all purpose flour

1 tsp baking powder

1 tsp baking soda

Pinch of coarse kosher salt

1 cup semi sweet mini chocolate chips

Pink Himalayan sea salt for sprinkling on top

Directions:

- In a large mixing bowl, using an electric mixer, cream together the butter and both sugars until light and fluffy (about 1-2 minutes). Add the eggs and continue to mix until just combined.
- Add the espresso powder and vanilla extract and continue to mix until smooth (you may need to scrape down the sides of the bowl to incorporate all of the espresso powder.
- In a separate small mixing bowl, combine the flour, baking soda, baking powder, and pinch of salt.
- Combine the flour mixture to the wet ingredients and mix until well combined.
- Fold in the mini chocolate chips.
- Using a Scoop #40 (1 ½ inches size), begin scooping out cookie balls onto a large baking sheet. (You will chill the dough before baking so there is no need to space the cookies out yet.)
- Once the dough is scooped out into pre-measured balls, sprinkle the tops with flakes of pink himalayan sea salt. Place the baking sheet in the refrigerator for 1 hour to chill. This allows the butter to set and reduce the cookies from spreading too much.
- Once the cookie dough is chilled, preheat the oven to 350 degrees Fahrenheit and prepare another baking sheet with parchment paper. Transfer about 10 cookies to the prepared baking sheet and place them accordingly with room to spread.
- Bake for 13-15 minutes or until golden brown.

Tips:

Best served slightly warm.

Store in an airtight container for up to 7 days.

☆☆☆☆☆

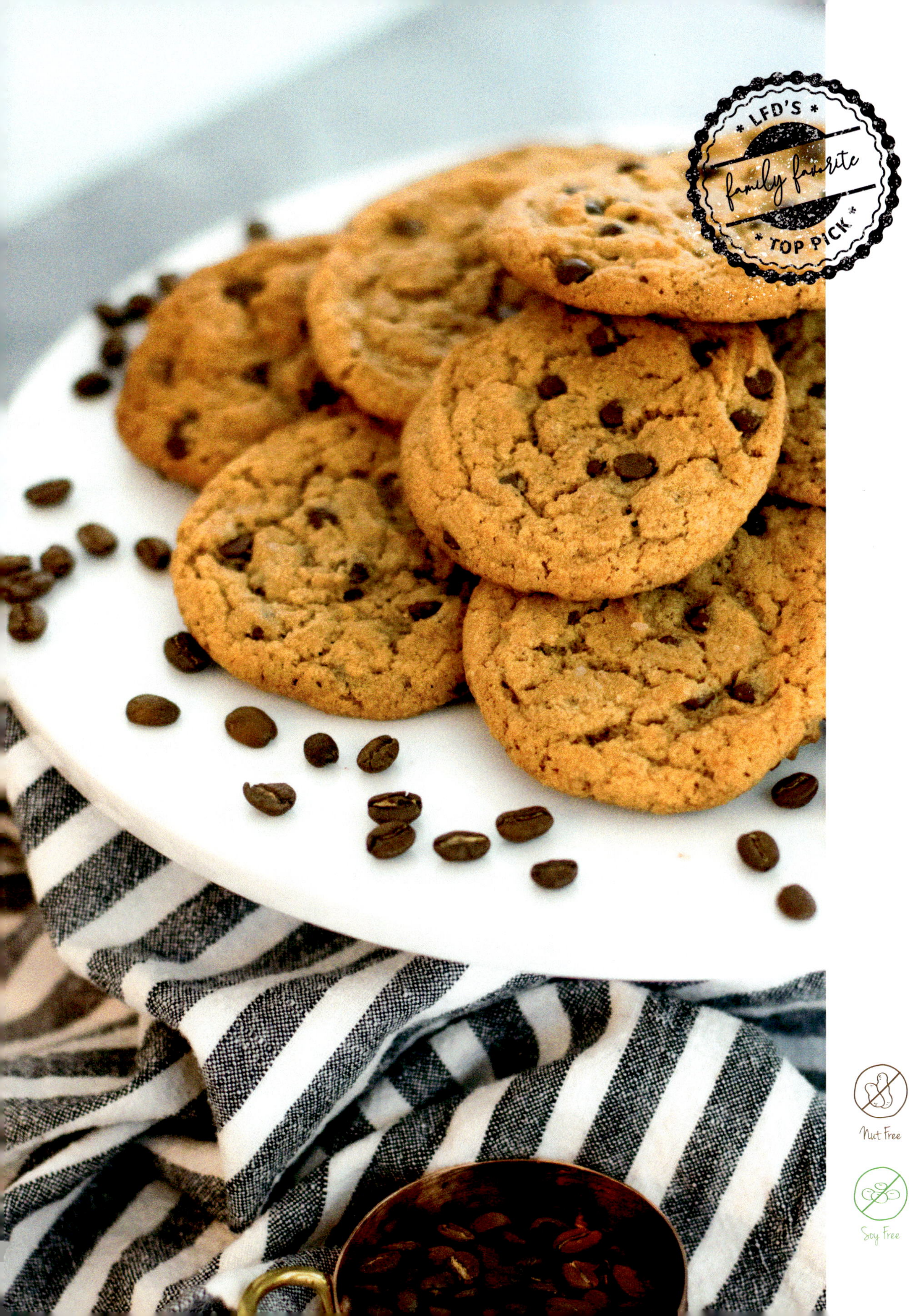

Nut Free

Soy Free

Chocolate Thumbprint Cookies

If you know my husband, you know we always keep a stash of chocolate somewhere in the house. I may not be the crazy chocolate lover in the family, but I do love to bake with chocolate because it makes him the happiest. You may already know about the health benefits of dark chocolate, but non-alkalized 100% naturally unsweetened cocoa powder has a few health benefits tricks up its sleeve as well. If you can find non-alkalized cocoa powder in the store, it contains flavanols, which can help reduce blood pressure and improve vascular and circulation function. Now, making these cookies with cocoa powder might not be a cure for your blood pressure, but I can guarantee happiness from the first delicious bite.

PREP TIME: 15 minutes

COOK TIME: 13 minutes

YIELDS: 12 cookies

Ingredients:

10 tbsp butter, softened

1 cup granulated sugar

1 large egg

1 tsp vanilla extract

1 cup all purpose flour

¾ cup 100% naturally unsweetened cocoa powder

1 tsp baking powder

Pinch of salt

Good quality Strawberry jam

Optional:
Confectioners' sugar to dust on top

Directions:

- Preheat the oven to 350 degrees Fahrenheit. Prepare a baking sheet with parchment paper.
- In a large mixing bowl, cream together the butter and sugar until light and fluffy (about 1-2 minutes). Next, add the egg and vanilla extract.
- In a separate mixing bowl, combine the flour, cocoa powder, baking powder, and pinch of salt.
- Combine the flour mixture with the wet ingredients and mix until well combined.
- Roll into 1 inch balls and place on a baking sheet. Using your thumb, press into the cookie ball in two directions making a heart shape in the middle.
- Bake for 10 minutes and pull from the oven. While the cookies are still warm, using a small spoon such as a ¼ tsp measuring spoon, press into the existing heart shape to create a deeper imprint (but not so deep as to touch the bottom of the cookie or break the cookie).
- Gently spoon the strawberry jam into the heart shape of each cookie. Place back in the oven for 3 minutes to set.

Optional: Once the cookies are cooled, dust the top with the confectioner's sugar. The confectioner's sugar will dissipate into the jam over several hours, and you'll be left with the heart shape.

Tip:

Store in an airtight container for up to 5-6 days.

☆☆☆☆☆

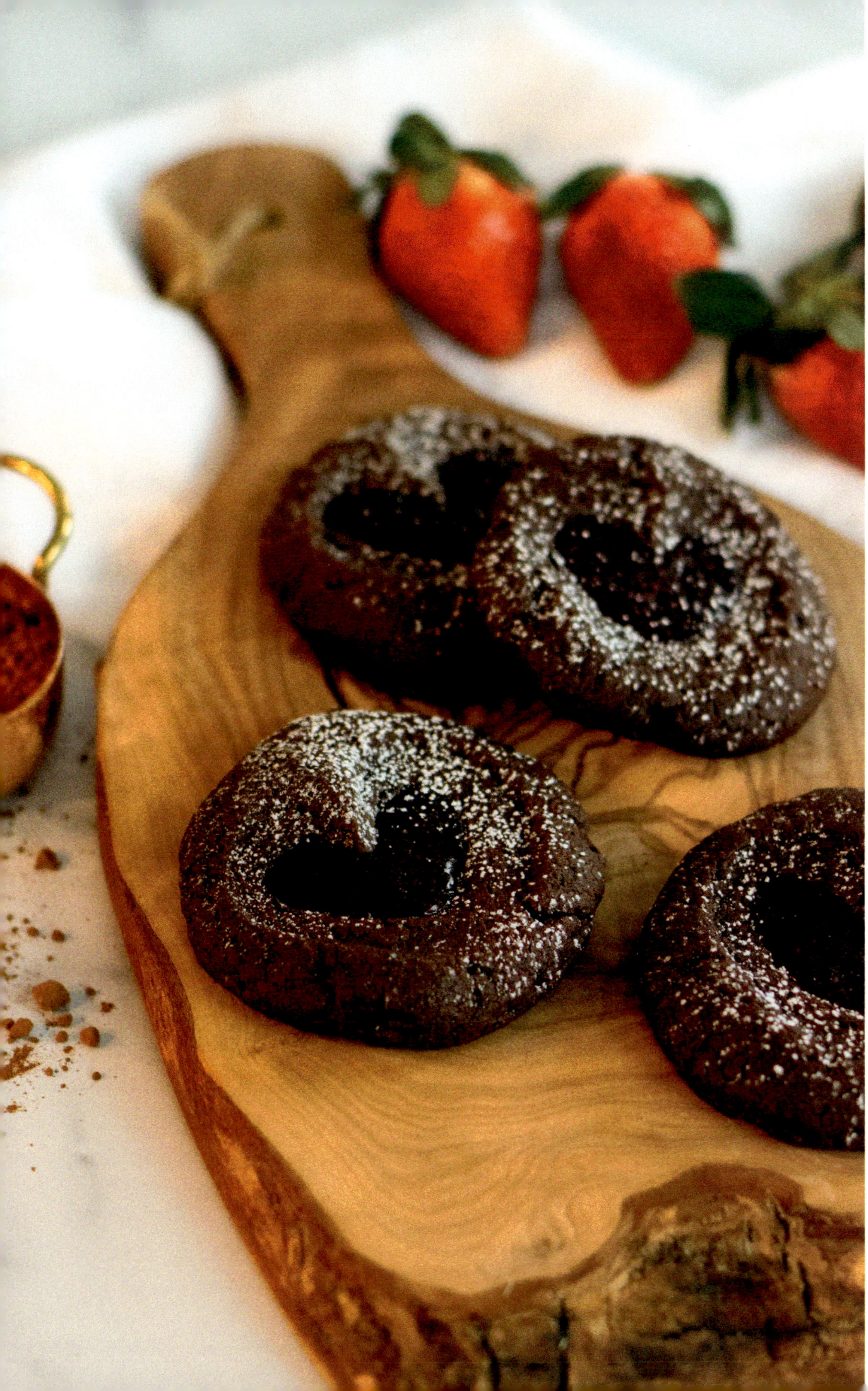

Nut Free

Soy Free

Dirty Bourbon Balls

If you could be a bourbon of choice, which one would you choose? I'm not exactly a straight bourbon lover, but I appreciate a slight note of bourbon in my desserts, especially when paired with chocolate. There's something strong and masculine about a good bourbon. From the earthy notes they possess, the deep aging tradition, and the gentlemen-like atmosphere it promotes- no two bourbons are the same. Among our family's favorite bourbons include Woodford Reserve™, Blanton's Single Barrel™, and Buffalo Trace™.
When making these bourbon balls, simply reduce the amount to 2-3 tbs if you prefer less bourbon taste.

PREP TIME: 45 minutes

CHILL TIME: 1+ hour

COOK TIME: No Bake

YIELDS: 35-40 cookies

Ingredients:

2 ½ cups finely crushed honey graham crackers

1 ¾ cup finely chopped pecans

1 cup semi sweet chocolate chips + ½ cup for drizzling on top

½ cup packed light brown sugar

¼ cup light corn syrup

¼ cup bourbon of choice

Pinch of salt

Directions:

- Prepare a large baking sheet with parchment paper.
- Using a food processor, finely chop the graham crackers until it resembles a coarse flour, set aside for later.
- Using a food processor, finely chop the pecans, set aside for later.
- In a large microwavable bowl, melt 1 cup of chocolate chips for 1-2 minutes in the microwave. Using a spatula, mix well until all the lumps are gone.
- Add the brown sugar, corn syrup, bourbon, and salt to the chocolate and stir to combine.
- Add the finely chopped pecans and finely crushed graham crackers to the chocolate mixture, stir to combine.
- Using a tablespoon, scoop out the dough and roll into individual balls. Place on the prepared baking sheet.
- Melt the remaining ½ cup chocolate chips in a glass measuring cup. Using a fork, mix together until all the lumps are gone. While the chocolate is still warm, drizzle over the bourbon balls.
- Place in the refrigerator to let set for at least 1 hour.

Tips:

Store in the fridge for up to 10 days. It can be stored in the freezer for later use as well.

When ready to serve, take it out of the fridge for several hours to bring it back to room temperature.

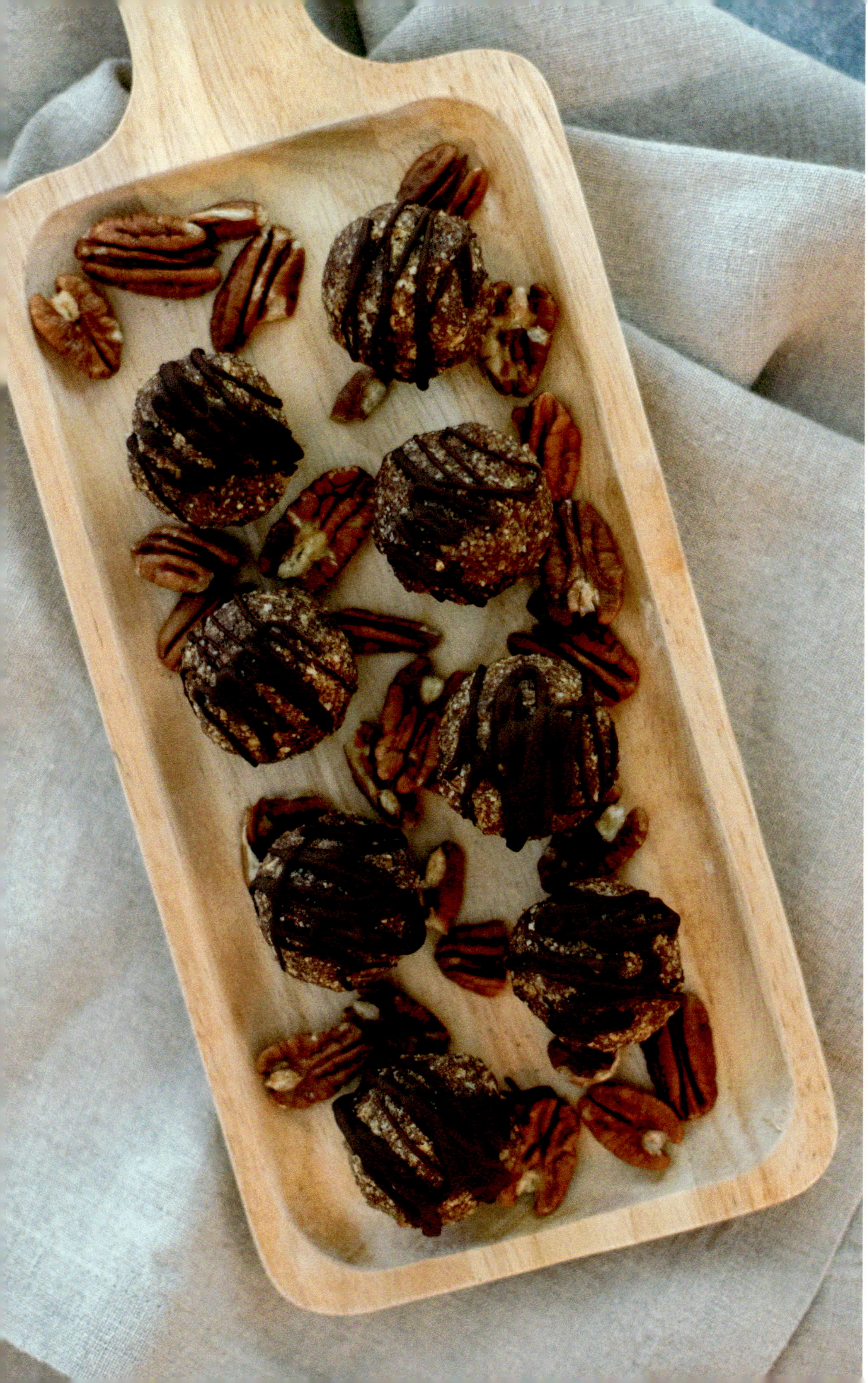

Egg Free

Dairy Free

Chocolate Peanut Butter Smash Cookies

Whether you choose to use almond butter or peanut butter in this recipe, it's bound to be delicious and loaded with some health benefits as well. Almond butter is our preferable ingredient in the Rackley house because of Justin's peanut allergy, and to be honest; I prefer almond butter to peanut butter any day. Almond butter is high in monounsaturated fats, which help to increase your HDL (good) cholesterol and drive down your LDL (bad) cholesterol. Almond butter also contains plenty of fiber, which is essential for gut motility, among many other processes. Lastly, almond butter contains vitamin E, calcium, magnesium, phosphorus, and manganese, which are necessary vitamins and nutrients for the body. So go ahead, pick your favorite (almond butter vs. peanut butter) and get smashin' and snackin' on these delicious cookies.

PREP TIME: 15 minutes

COOK TIME: 13 minutes

YIELDS: 19 cookies

Ingredients:

10 tbsp butter, softened

1 cup granulated sugar

1 large egg

1 tsp vanilla extract

1 cup all purpose flour

¾ cup 100% naturally unsweetened cocoa powder

1 tsp baking powder

Pinch of salt

¾ cup creamy style peanut butter (or almond butter)

Directions:

- Preheat the oven to 350 degrees Fahrenheit. Prepare two baking sheets with parchment paper.
- In a large mixing bowl, cream together the butter and sugar until light and fluffy (about 1-2 minutes). Next, add the egg and vanilla extract.
- In a separate mixing bowl, combine the flour, cocoa powder, baking powder, and pinch of salt.
- Combine the flour mixture to the wet ingredients and mix until well combined.
- Fold in the peanut butter using a spatula, turning the dough only a few times to allow for the difference in colors (peanut butter and chocolate) to maintain visibility.
- Using a Scoop #40 (1 ½ inches size), scoop out the portioned cookie dough onto the prepared baking sheets (cookies will not spread, so feel free to space cookies closer together).
- Bake for 13 minutes.
- While the cookies are still warm, use a fork to gently smash the cookies in 2 different directions like a traditional peanut butter cookie.

Tip:

Store in an airtight container for up to 7 days.

☆☆☆☆☆

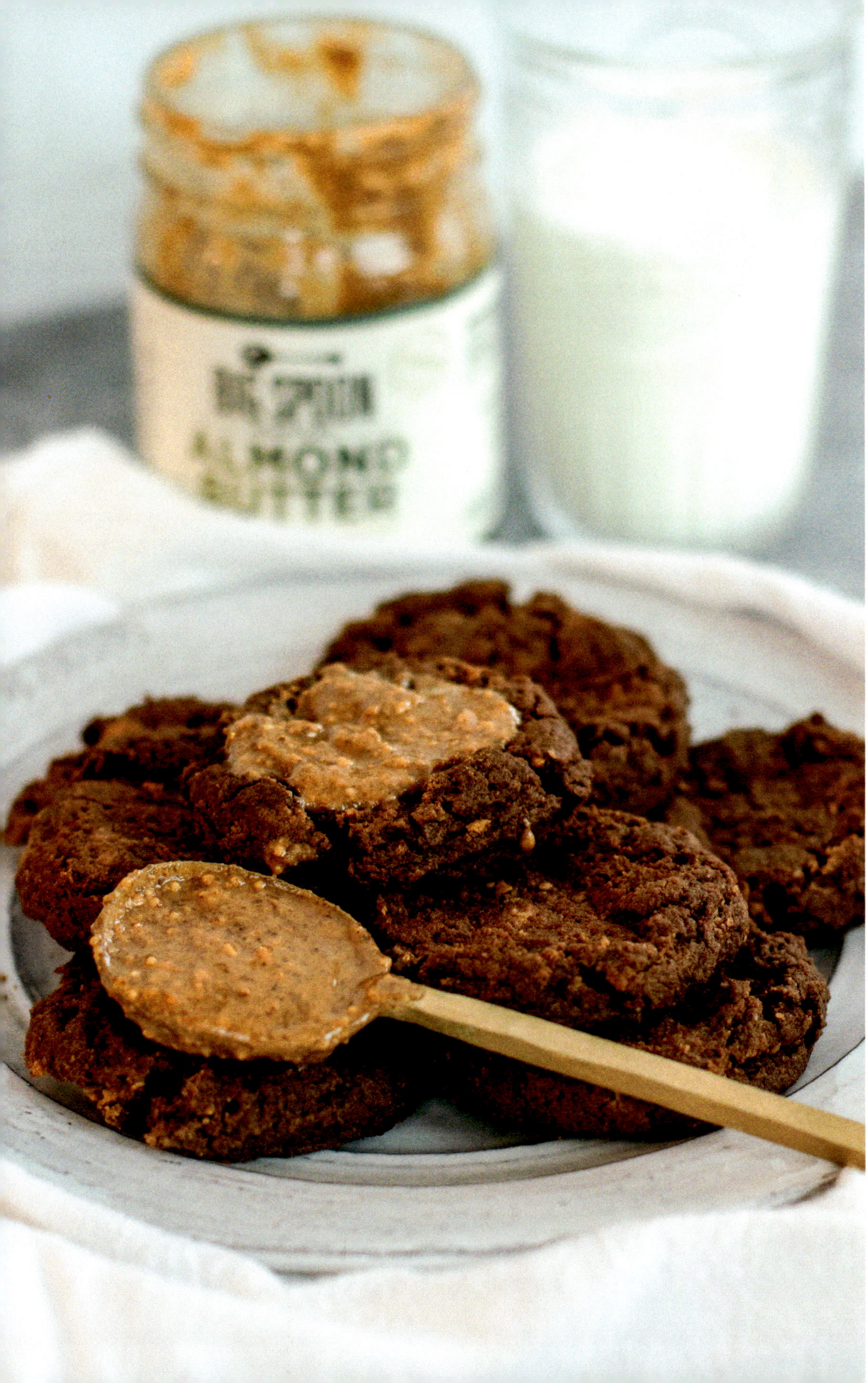

Soy Free

Classic Snickerdoodle Ice Cream Sandwich Cookies

When the summer temperature rises, and there's no escape from the heat, these cookies need to be on the menu. The soft snickerdoodle cookie and the cold ice cream delight make the little extra time required to prep these sandwiches so worth it. My tip of advice is to make everything ahead of time, and when the kids (or you) start asking for dessert, it's as simple as unwrapping the ice cream and staying mess-free. Ice cream sandwiches are another timeless summertime treat that I couldn't leave out of this book. Sure, you could go buy some at the store, but there's always something sweeter about your favorite vanilla ice cream sandwiched between warm homemade cookies.

PREP TIME: 25 minutes

COOK TIME: 15-17 minutes

YIELDS: 8 sandwiches or 16 cookies

Ingredients:

½ cup butter, softened

1 cup granulated sugar

3 large egg yolks

1 ½ cup all purpose flour

1 tsp baking soda

1 tsp ground cinnamon

1 tsp cream of tartar

½ tsp salt

½ cup granulated sugar

1 tbsp ground cinnamon

2 frozen pints of your favorite vanilla ice cream

Directions:

- Preheat the oven to 350 degrees Fahrenheit. Prepare 2 baking sheets with parchment paper.
- In a large mixing bowl, cream together the butter and sugar until light and fluffy (about 2-3 minutes). Add the egg yolks and mix until just combined.
- In a separate mixing bowl, whisk together the flour, baking soda, cinnamon, cream of tartar, and salt.
- Combine the flour mixture with the wet ingredients and mix until well combined.
- In a separate small bowl, combine the additional ½ cup sugar and 1 tbsp of cinnamon.
- Roll the cookie dough into 1 inch balls. Continue to roll the cookie balls in the sugar mixture to cover well and place them on the prepared baking sheets.
- Bake for 15-16 minutes. The cookies will not appear to be done, considering the cracking gives way to gooey dough; however, they cool/harden fast after being taken out of the oven. The key to ice cream sandwiches is creating a soft cookie to sink your teeth into. Harder cookies cause the ice cream to squish/slide out.
- While the cookies are baking, cut the ice cream molds. Place the ice cream pints horizontally on a cutting board. Using a sharp serrated bread knife, cut through the pints of ice cream to create circular rounds. I found cutting 5 rounds of ice cream molds (per pint) was the perfect ratio of cookie to ice cream.

Tips:

Best served immediately after baking while the ice cream is still frozen.

Prepping the cookies beforehand and pre-cutting the ice cream pints works well if preparing for a gathering or party. Simply store the pre-cut ice cream rounds in the freezer and the cookies in an airtight container until ready to serve.

☆☆☆☆☆

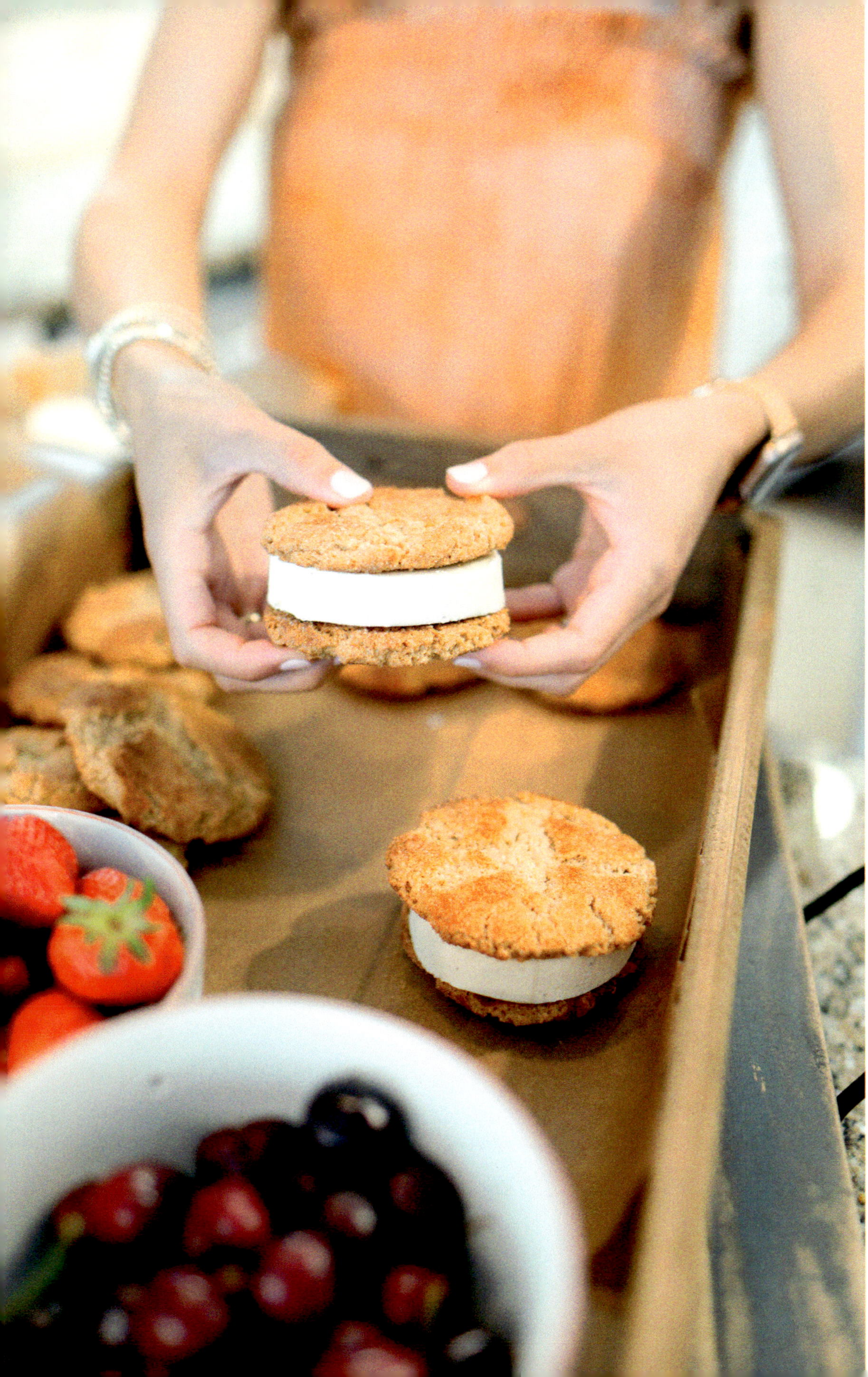

Nut Free

Soy Free

Not So Traditional Oatmeal Chocolate Chip Cookies

Looking for a simple yet incredibly delicious cookie staple to have on hand? You have officially landed on the right page and found it. Although simple might be underrated in today's society, we can't shake the truth that sometimes simpler is better. There is beauty in simplicity, and these cookies are tried and true examples of that. When asking many of my followers what they wished to see in this cookie cookbook, many of them replied with an unexpected answer, "Oatmeal Chocolate Chip Cookies." I guess there is something to be said about that; tradition will always reign.

Although these are oatmeal chocolate chip cookies, they don't have an overpowering oatmeal-like taste. You get the best of both worlds when you sink your teeth and heart into this warm freshly-baked cookie. Partly tasting like a traditional chocolate chip cookie and partly tasting like oatmeal, this cookie soothes the craving for both at one time. So, maybe you can have the cookie and eat it too?

PREP TIME: 10 minutes

COOK TIME: 17 minutes

YIELDS: 16-17 cookies

Ingredients:

½ cup butter, softened

1 cup packed light brown sugar

1 large egg

1 tsp pure vanilla extract

1 ¼ cup all purpose flour

¾ cup quick oats

1 tsp baking powder

½ tsp salt

Directions:

- Preheat the oven to 325 degrees Fahrenheit and prepare a baking sheet with parchment paper.
- Cream together the butter and sugar until light and fluffy. Add the egg and vanilla and continue to beat until incorporated.
- In a separate bowl, combine the flour, oatmeal, baking powder, and salt. Whisk until incorporated.
- Slowly add the flour mixture to the butter mixture (half at a time) and mix until just combined and no dry flour is visible.
- Begin rolling dough into 1" balls and place on the prepared baking sheet.
- Bake for 17 minutes .

Tip:

Store in an airtight container for up to 6 days.

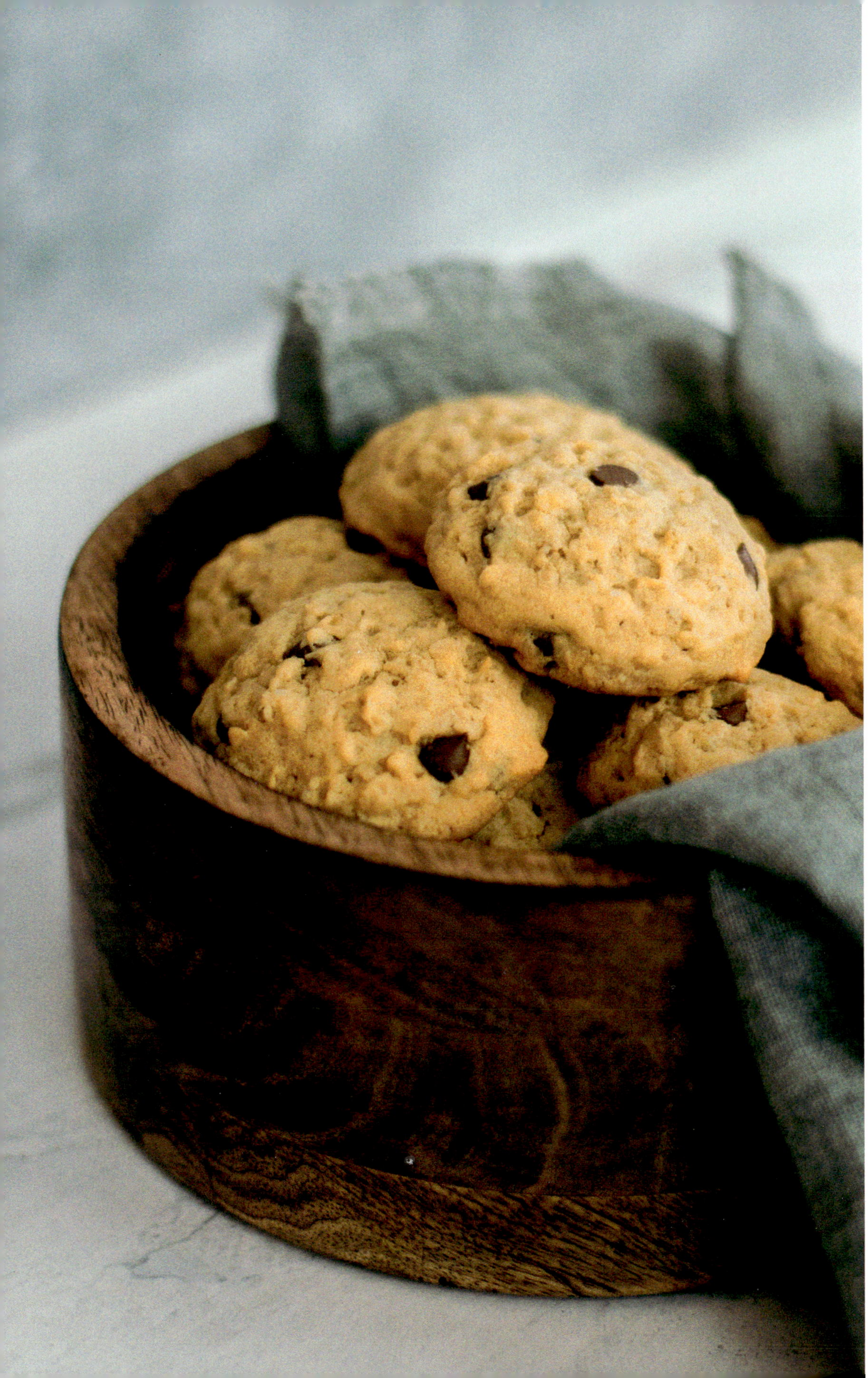

Nut Free

Soy Free

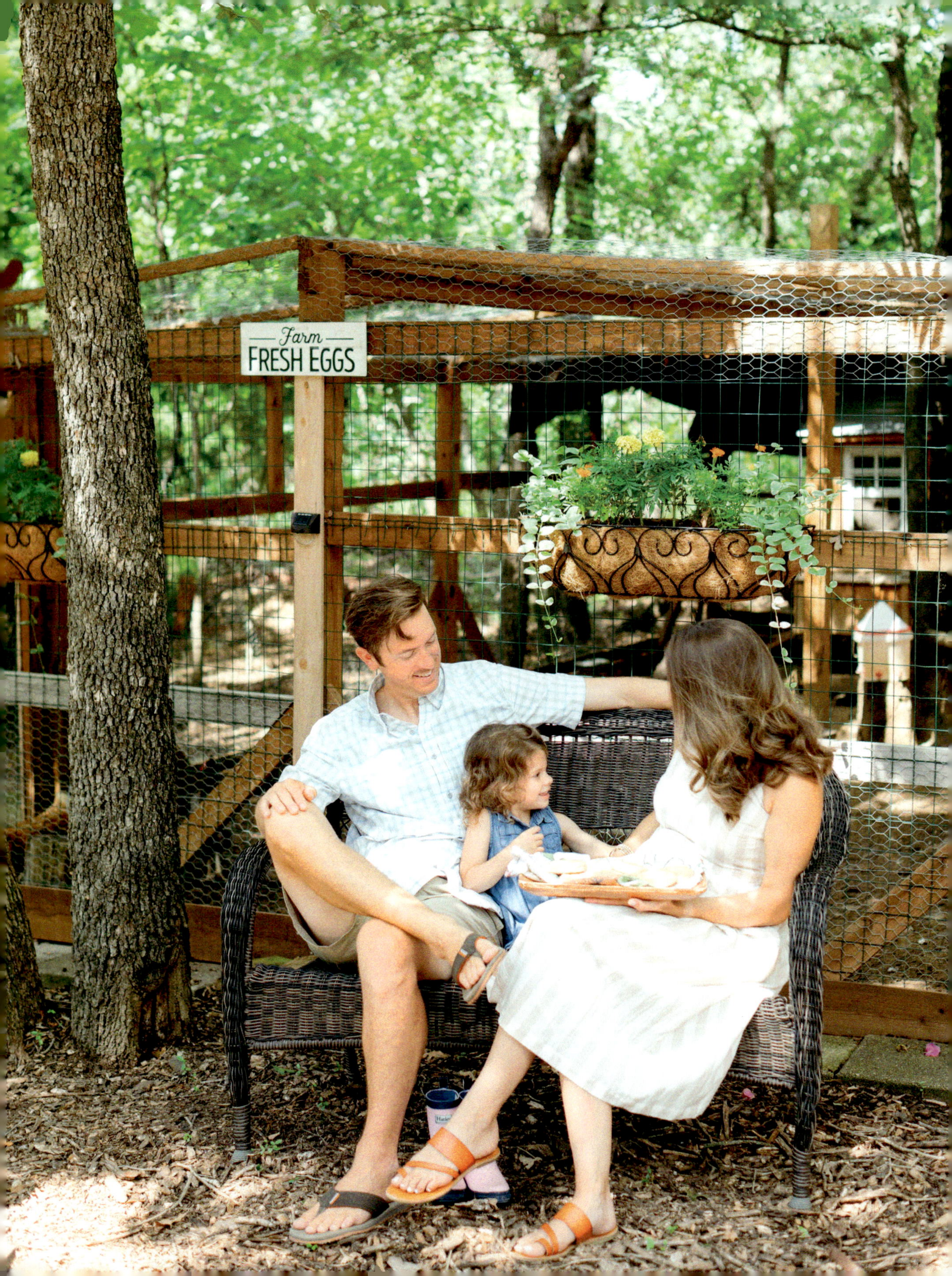
Farm
FRESH EGGS

Our tried and true family Cookie favorites

- Pumpkin Spice Snickerdoodle with Coconut Cream Frosting
- Locked and Loaded Cowboy Cookies *(Mimi's Pick)*
- Brownie Cream Filled Sandwich Cookies
- Down-To-Earth Woodsman Cookies *(Justin's Pick)*
- Triple Layer Threat Chocolate Chip Cookies
- The OG Gingerbread Snickerdoodle Cookies *(Justin's Pick)*
- Simple Christmas Gingerbread Cookies

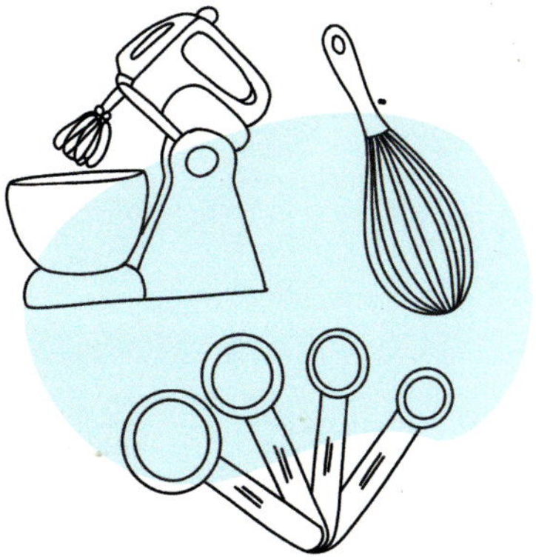

This section contains most of our family's original favorite cookie recipes. These are the recipes that started it all. From the very beginning, back when I hadn't even owned a mixer of my own, nor did I know what a pastry cutter was, I found my passion for baking and creating recipes in the kitchen that we would enjoy for years to come. Creating recipes and experimenting with ingredients has always interested me, and I am so thankful to have a husband who supports me endlessly in this area. From my first attempt at homemade pancakes that turned out pasty white and tasted like play dough (I'll never forget the baking soda/powder again) to creating some of our favorite traditions in the kitchen, I've had my fair share of baking failures. However, because of these failures, I am proud to share my successful tried and true favorites with you in this section.

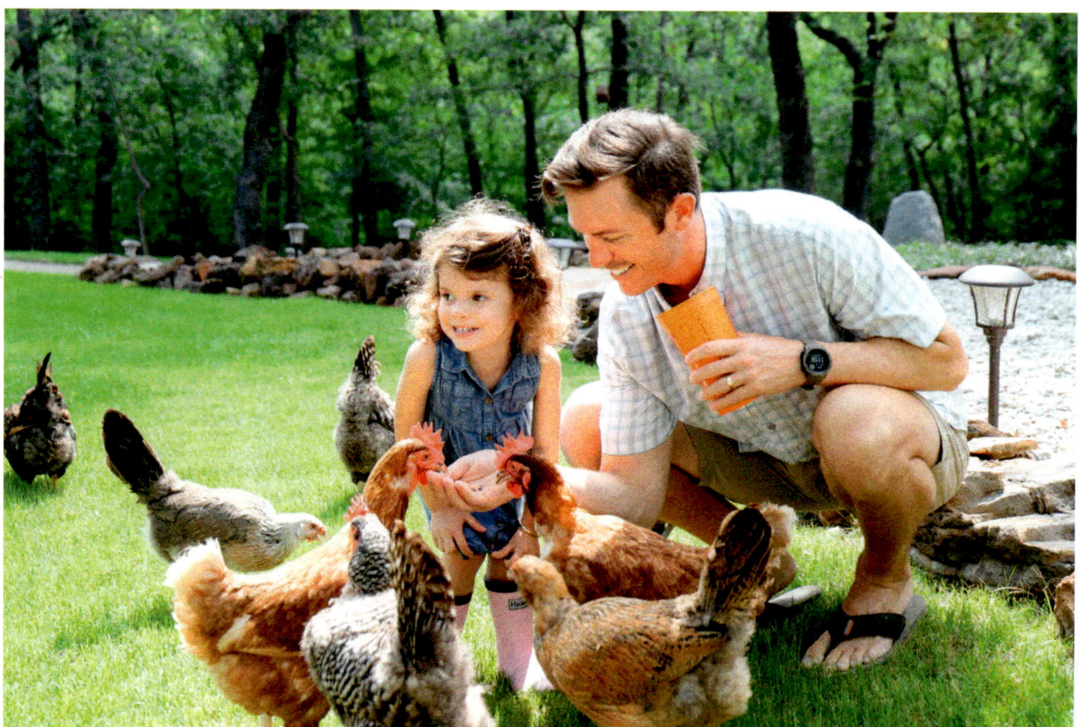

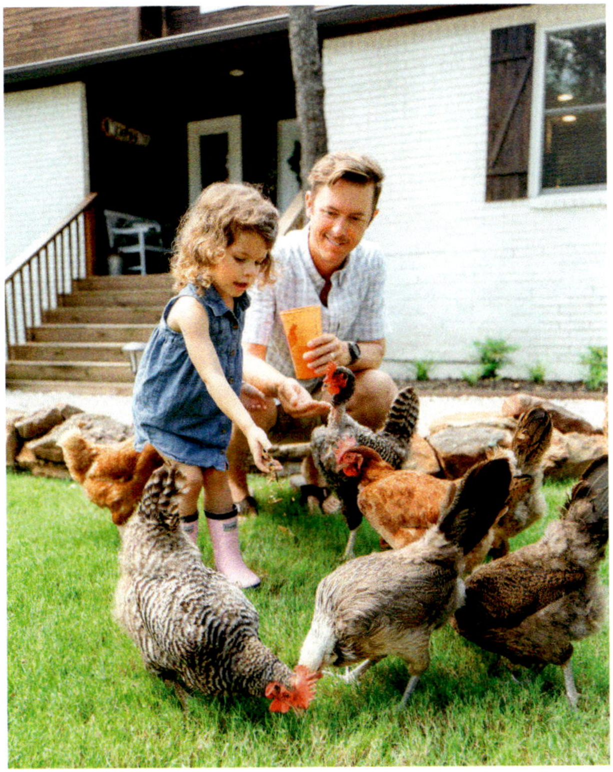

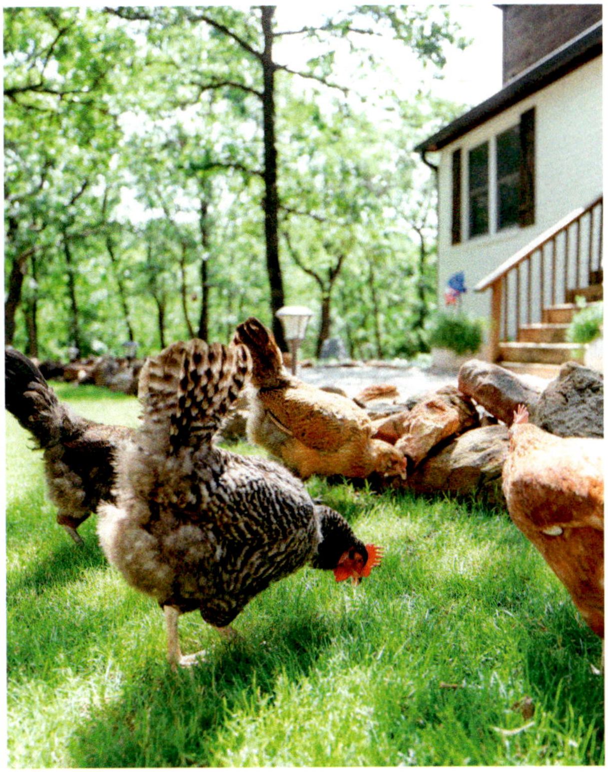

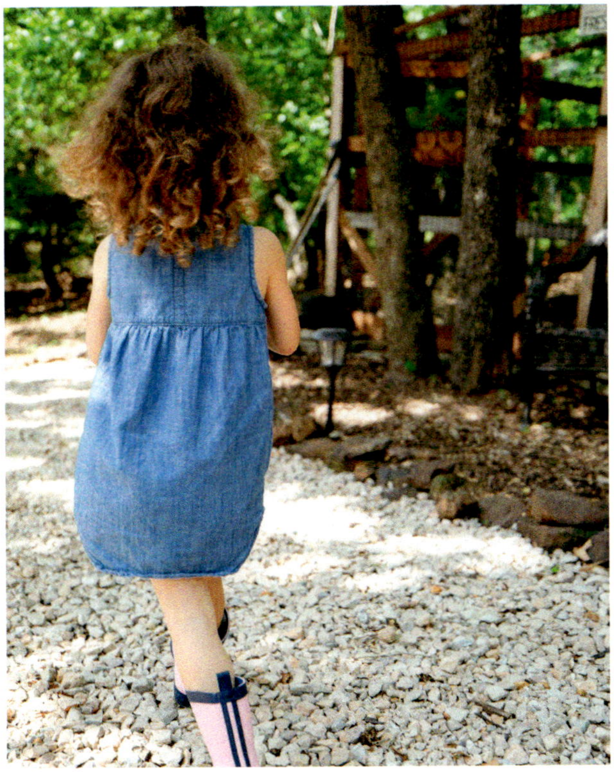

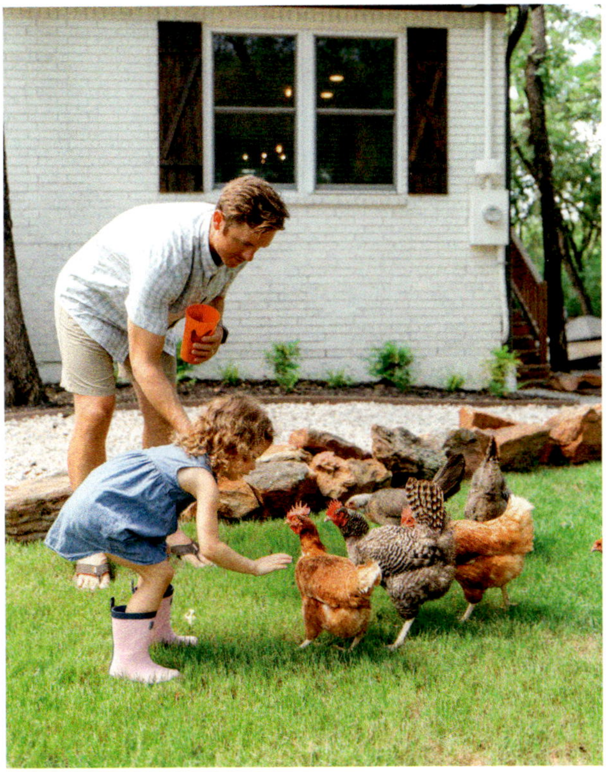

Pumpkin Spice Snickerdoodle with Coconut Cream Frosting

A fall twist on my OG gingerbread snickerdoodle cookies, these cookies were made for the fall baking season. The smell of them baking alone will cause you to think about front porch pumpkins, cozy plaid, chilly weather, and all things October. It's a wonderful time of the year when pumpkin spice items hit the shelves in your local grocery store; however, you don't have to wait all year to enjoy these sweet pumpkin treats. The additional coconut cream frosting creates a simple, sweet layer without overpowering the pumpkin spices you know and love. I think one of the best parts of this recipe is that you'll have some leftover pumpkin puree, which I always use as an excuse to make pumpkin bread or pumpkin pancakes the next day.

PREP TIME: 25 minutes

COOK TIME: 15 minutes

YIELDS: 20 cookies

Ingredients:

FOR THE COOKIES

¾ cup butter, softened

1 cup granulated sugar

1 large egg

¼ cup pumpkin puree (not pumpkin pie filling)

2 ½ cup all purpose flour

½ tsp ground nutmeg

½ tsp ground cloves

2 tsp pumpkin pie spice

¾ tsp ground cinnamon

1 tsp baking soda

Pinch of salt

⅓ cup granulated sugar

FOR THE FROSTING

13-14 oz can of coconut cream chilled for about 24 hours (note this is coconut cream, not coconut milk. Make sure it is chilled, not frozen when getting ready to use for the frosting)

½ cup granulated sugar

1 tsp pure vanilla extract

1 tsp cream of tartar

Directions:

- Preheat the oven to 350 degrees Fahrenheit. Prepare 2 baking sheets with parchment paper.
- In a large mixing bowl, cream together the butter and sugar until light and fluffy (about 2-3 minutes). Add the egg and pumpkin puree and mix until combined.
- In a separate mixing bowl, whisk together the flour, nutmeg, cloves, pumpkin pie spice, cinnamon, baking soda, and salt.
- Combine the flour mixture (half at a time) with the wet ingredients and mix until well combined.
- In a separate small bowl, pour the additional 1/3 cup sugar.
- Roll the cookie dough into 1-1 ½ inch balls. Continue to roll the cookie balls in the sugar to cover well and place on the prepared baking sheets.
- Bake for 15 minutes.
- While the cookies are baking, begin making the coconut cream frosting.
- Open and pour the can of coconut cream into a mixing bowl (if chilled correctly, the cream should be separate from the liquid. Discard the liquid.) Using an electric mixer, beat the coconut cream, sugar, vanilla, and cream of tartar until smooth and creamy.
- When cookies are done baking and cooling, begin frosting the tops of the cookies with an icing spatula.

Optional: Add a second layer of frosting once the first layer has set. The frosting will not fully harden but will set slightly once cooled. Photos shown have two layers of frosting.

Tip:

Store in the fridge for 5-6 days.

☆☆☆☆☆

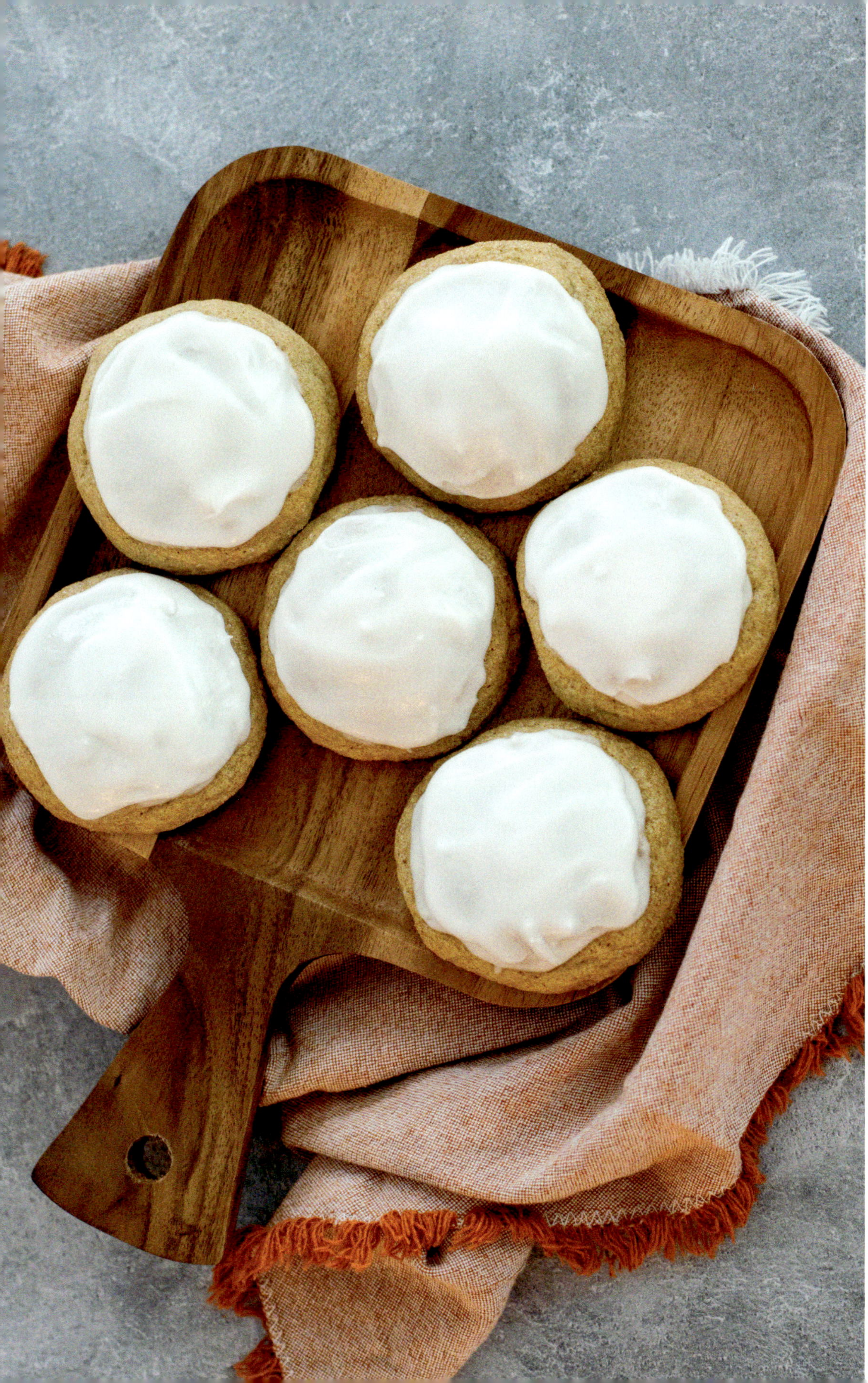

Dairy Free Frosting

Nut Free

Soy Free

Locked and Loaded Cowboy Cookies

These cookies made it into our family's top five favorite cookies. If you're not familiar, cowboy cookies have become more popular in recent years, mostly due to Laura Bush's cowboy cookie recipe that won the First Lady Bake-Off in 2000. These days, most cowboy cookies contain relatively the same ingredients, including oats, pecans, coconut, and chocolate. However, I figured I would keep the pile going by adding an additional ingredient (pretzels) to make sure these were as loaded as they could possibly get. Make room and clear the counter space because these cookies are absolutely locked and loaded with ALL the fixin's.

PREP TIME: 20 minutes

COOK TIME: 12-13 minutes

YIELDS: 20 cookies

Ingredients:

1 cup butter, softened

1 cup packed light brown sugar

½ cup granulated sugar

2 large eggs + 1 large egg yolk, room temperature

2 tsp pure vanilla extract

1 ½ cup all purpose flour

1 tsp baking soda

1 ½ tsp ground cinnamon

Pinch of salt

3 cups old fashioned rolled oats

½ cup shredded coconut (either sweetened or unsweetened works well)

½ cup coarsely chopped pecans

1 cup semi-sweet chocolate chips

½ cup coarsely chopped pretzel sticks

Topping: Pink Himalayan salt

Topping: Additional shredded coconut

Directions:

- Preheat the oven to 350 degrees Fahrenheit. Prepare two baking sheets with parchment paper.
- In a large mixing bowl, cream together the butter and both sugars until light and fluffy (about 2-3 minutes). Add the eggs and vanilla extract and continue to beat until incorporated.
- In a separate mixing bowl, whisk together the flour, baking soda, ground cinnamon, and salt.
- Combine the flour mixture with the wet ingredients and mix until combined.
- Fold in the rolled oats, shredded coconut, pecans, chocolate chips, and pretzel sticks until evenly distributed.
- Roll into 2 inch balls (or use a 2" ice cream scoop) and place on the baking sheets with room to spread. You will have excess dough. I reused one of my baking sheets once the first batch was done cooking.
- Bake for 12-13 minutes or until the edges have slightly browned. The middle will still appear to be slightly undercooked, but they will set a few minutes after being taken out of the oven.
- Sprinkle with additional shredded coconut and pink Himalayan salt while still warm.

Tip:

Store in an airtight container for up to 1 week.

☆☆☆☆☆

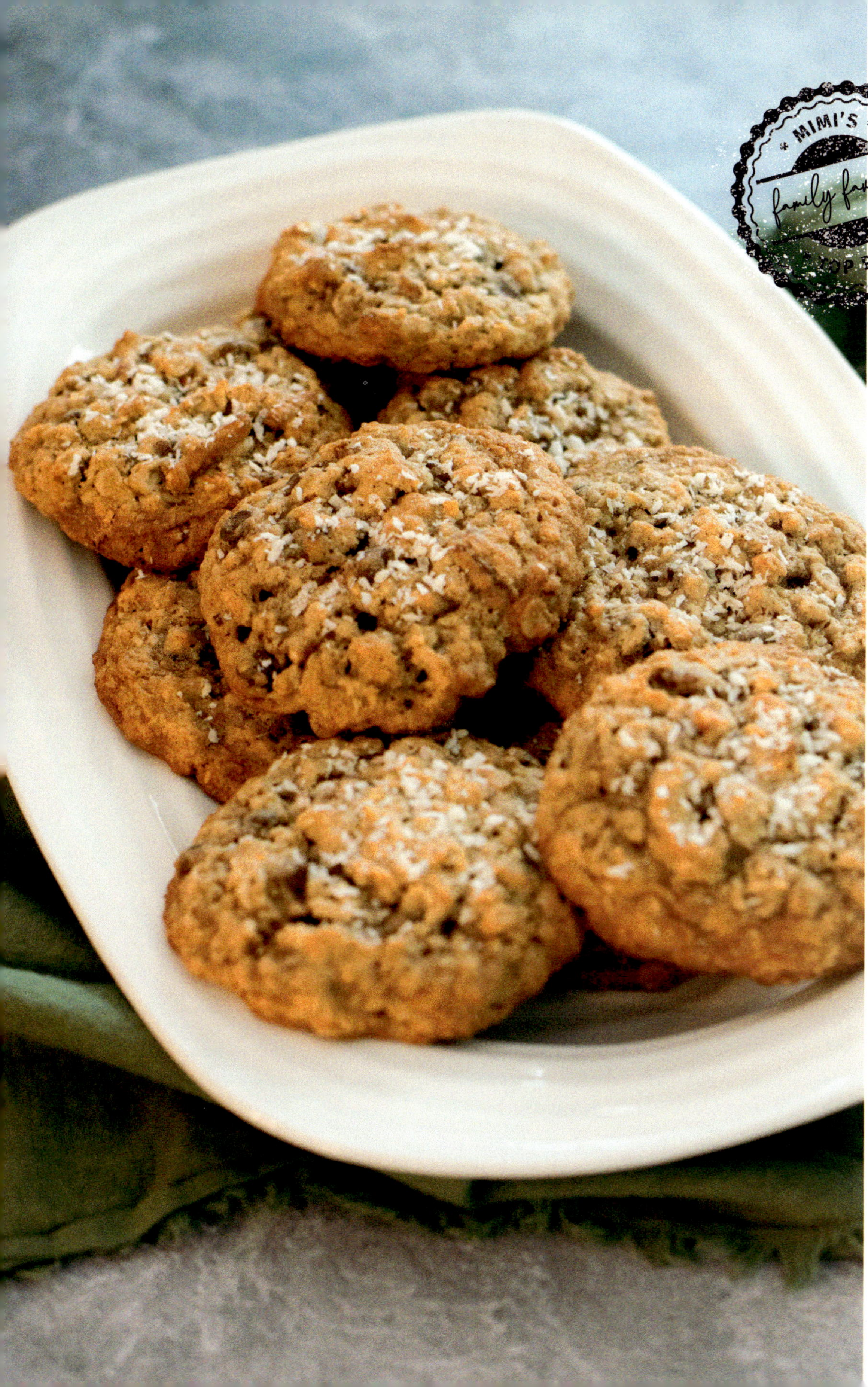

Soy Free

Brownie Cream Filled Sandwich Cookies

Have a bite of these cookies, and let me take you back to when Little Debbie™ snacks were in every kids' lunch box, and nobody thought anything different about it. But, of course, these days are a little different. These days we aim to make healthier choices daily, and I wouldn't dream of placing a Little Debbie™ snack in my toddler's lunch box. However, that's not to say she hasn't taken a bite or two (or more) of these cream-filled treats. Sometimes in life, dessert is the answer, and I think homemade dessert is the best answer. One of my most loved cookie recipes, these will not disappoint. Whether you bake them up for yourself or a gathering of people, I guarantee you will have people asking for more.

PREP TIME: 25 minutes

CHILL TIME: 20 minutes

COOK TIME: 10 minutes

YIELDS: 27 sandwich cookies

Ingredients:

FOR THE COOKIES

½ cup butter, softened

1 cup granulated sugar

2 large eggs

1 tsp pure vanilla extract

½ cup 100% naturally unsweetened cocoa powder

¾ cup all purpose flour

1 tsp baking soda

Pinch of salt

FOR THE FROSTING

2 cups confectioner's sugar

1 ½ tsp pure vanilla extract

½ cup butter, softened

1 tbsp milk

Directions:

- Preheat the oven to 325 degrees Fahrenheit. Prepare 2 baking sheets with parchment paper.
- In a large mixing bowl, cream together the butter and sugar until light and fluffy (about 2-3 minutes). Add the eggs and vanilla and mix until combined.
- In a separate mixing bowl, whisk together the cocoa powder, flour, baking soda, and salt.
- Combine the flour mixture with the wet ingredients and mix until well-combined.
- Chill for about 20 minutes in the refrigerator.
- Using a Scoop #100 (or tablespoon), drop the cookies onto the prepared baking sheet. The cookie dough will be slightly tricky to work with and hard to shape with your hands alone. Using a kitchen tool and the drop method will provide the best results.
- Bake for 10 minutes and let cool.
- While the cookies are baking, begin making the cream filling.
- Using an electric mixer, combine the frosting ingredients together and whip until smooth and creamy (about 3-4 minutes). If your confectioner's sugar creates lumps or the frosting is not smooth, add another 1-2 tsp of milk.
- After the cookies have completely cooled, begin assembling them. Using an icing spatula, spread the cream filling on the bottom of one cookie and place a matching size cookie on top to create a sandwich cookie. Repeat with the remaining cookies.
- Serve freshly made.

Tips:

It can be stored in the fridge for up to one week.
Then, when serving, take them out of the refrigerator in time to let them come to room temperature.

☆☆☆☆☆

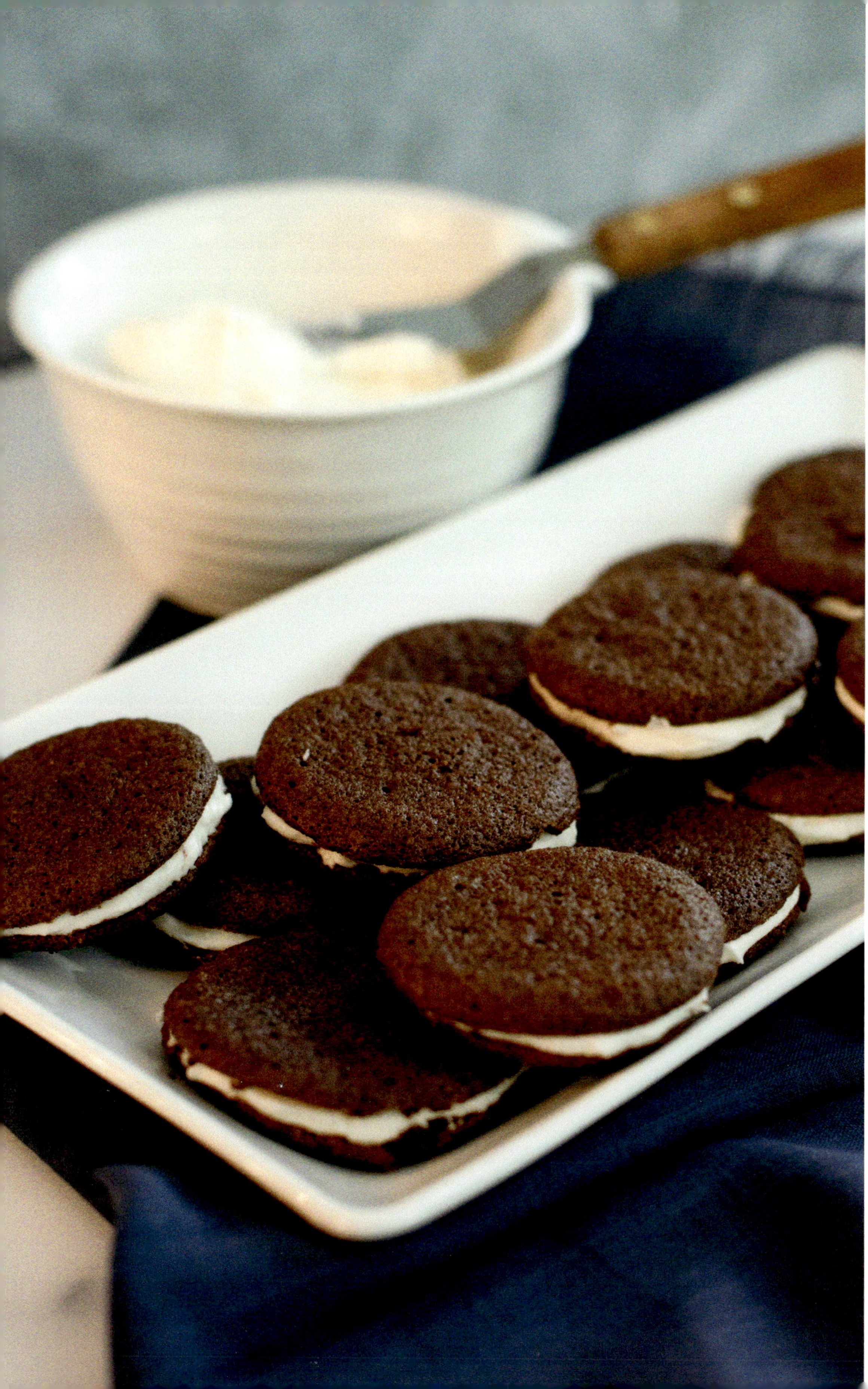

Nut Free

Soy Free

Down-To-Earth Woodsman Cookies

My Ode to all the woodsmen out there.

My husband, Justin, is an avid outdoorsman who lives and breathes the fresh air that comes with fishing, hunting, camping, you name it. He loves being up close and personal with nature, making it one of his life goals to survive entirely on his own in the wilderness. So you can imagine his preferences for decor, colors, tastes, and overall life theme always includes some sort of woodsman vibe. When we were first dating, I swear he dressed up a few times but now that we're happily married, his wardrobe consists of nothing but outdoors-ready pants and jackets in various shades of green and brown.

Justin designed this cookie by picking out certain ingredients he knew would pair well with his outdoor lifestyle. From the earthy taste of pecans to the pungent smell of rum, the cinnamon and anise create a vibe all on their own. Imagine yourself settled by the campfire, your long day hiking through the woods has come to a rest, and you're winding down by your cozy campsite.

Take a bite into these cookies, and you'll be transported into a woodsman's way of life.

PREP TIME: 20 minutes

COOK TIME: 10-12 minutes

YIELDS: 18 cookies

Ingredients:

½ cup butter, softened

½ cup packed light brown sugar

½ cup granulated sugar

1 large egg

1 tsp pure vanilla extract

1 tsp rum extract

1 ½ cup all purpose flour

1 cup ground pecans

1 tsp baking soda

1 tsp baking powder

1 tsp ground cinnamon

1 tsp anise

18 large pecan halves for the topping

Directions:

PREP: Using a food processor, finely chop the pecans.

- Preheat the oven to 350 degrees Fahrenheit. Prepare a baking sheet with parchment paper.
- In a large mixing bowl, cream the butter and both sugars together until light and fluffy (about 1-2 minutes). Next, add the egg, vanilla extract, and rum extract.
- In a separate mixing bowl, combine the flour, ground pecans, baking soda, baking powder, ground cinnamon, and anise.
- Combine the flour mixture with the wet ingredients and mix until well combined.
- Roll into 1 inch balls (or use a 1" ice cream scoop) and place on a baking sheet with room to spread.
- Bake for 8 minutes and take out of the oven
- Taking the large pecan halves, nestle one halve in the center of each cookie. Place back in the oven to continue baking for another 2-3 minutes or until golden brown, and slight crackings appear on the surface.
- Once the cookies are done baking, nestle the center pecan a little deeper to ensure they don't fall out later during storage.

Tip:

Store in an airtight container for up to 1 week.

☆☆☆☆☆

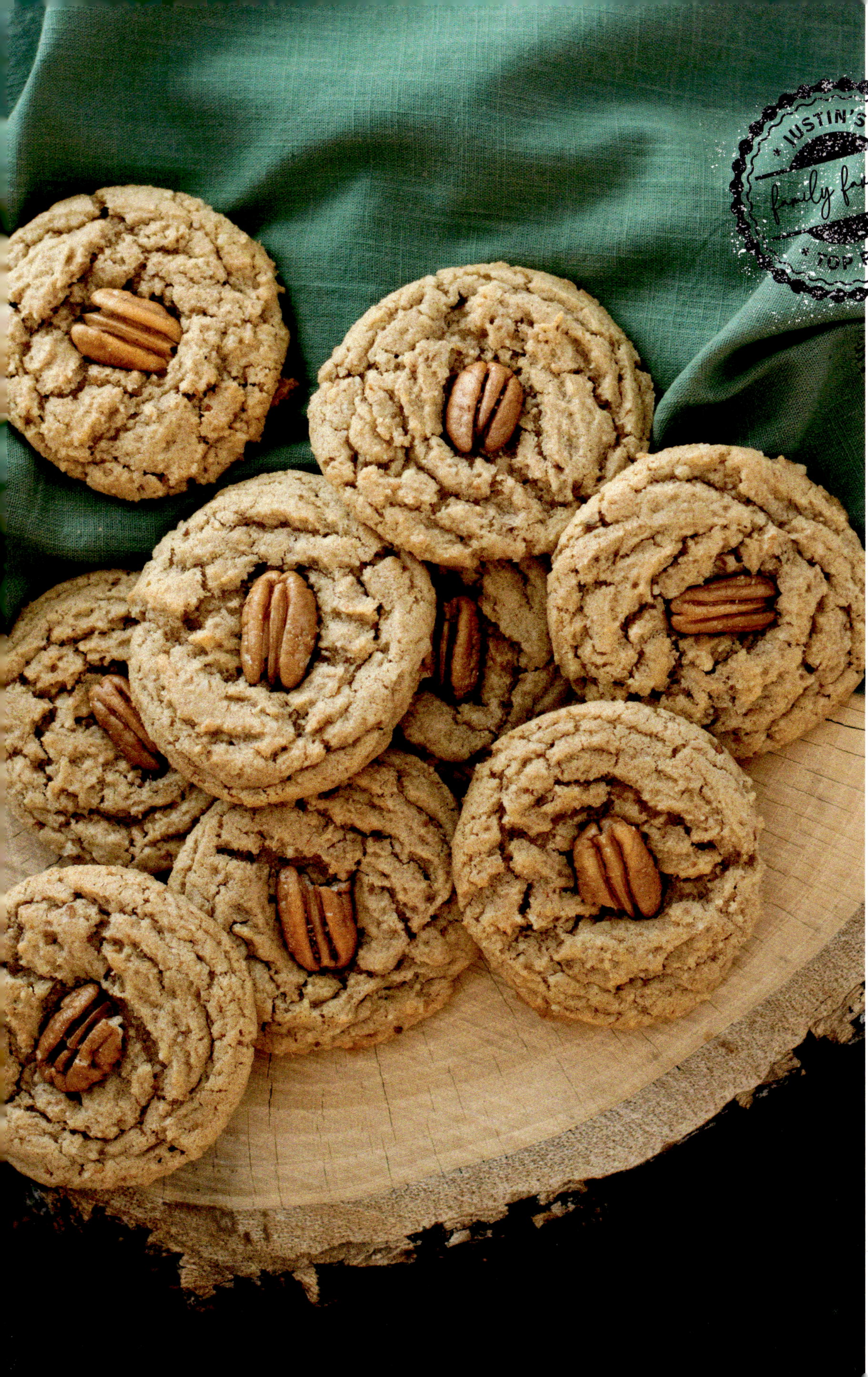

Soy Free

Triple Layer Threat Chocolate Chip Cookies
aka: Thousand layer chocolate chip cookies

One of the first cookie recipes I ever made for my husband, Justin. When we were first married, I took my role in the kitchen very seriously and always tried out new recipes, especially desserts, because my guy has the biggest sweet tooth you've ever seen. It's the way to his heart, and I learned this very early on. These cookies are truly a labor of love and not for the impatient baker. The number of steps to follow and layers to create make these cookies one of the hardest in my book. However, the finished product and the smile that comes after the first bite are always so worth it to me. So, if you're looking for something special, a cookie to celebrate a worthy accomplishment, you've landed on the right page. Just be patient, stay the course, and you'll have cookie masterpieces at the end.

PREP TIME: 30 minutes

CHILL TIME: 30+ minutes

COOK TIME: 12 minutes

YIELDS: 28-30 cookies

Ingredients:

1 cup butter, softened

¾ cup packed light brown sugar

¾ cup granulated sugar

4 large egg yolks + 1 whipped egg for glazing on top

1 tsp pure vanilla extract

2 ½ cup all purpose flour

1 tsp baking soda

Pinch of salt

1 cup dark chocolate chips

1 cup semi-sweet chocolate chips

Tip:

Store in an airtight container for up to one week.

☆☆☆☆☆

Directions:

- Preheat the oven to 375 degrees Fahrenheit. Prepare two baking sheets with parchment paper.
- Using a food processor, combine both the dark chocolate chips and the semi-sweet chocolate chips together. Pulse until the chips are reduced half in size but not powdered (about 1 minute) set chocolate crumbles aside for later.
- In a large mixing bowl, cream together the butter and both sugars until light and fluffy (about 2-3 minutes). Add the egg yolks two at a time and mix. Next, add the vanilla and mix until just combined. Do not overmix
- In a separate mixing bowl, whisk together the flour, baking soda, and salt.
- Combine the flour mixture with the wet ingredients and mix until well combined.
- Separate the dough into three equal portions and chill for about 30+ minutes in the refrigerator.
- Once the dough has chilled, lightly flour your work surface and begin rolling out the first portion of dough until about 1/3" thick. Taking 1/3 of the chocolate crumbles, spread them out evenly on the rolled dough.
- Taking the second chilled dough portion, place it on a large piece of lightly floured parchment paper. Repeat the same steps of rolling it out about 1/3" thick. Carefully transfer the rolled dough on top of the 1st layer with the chocolate crumbles.
- Repeat by taking another 1/3 of the chocolate crumbles and spreading it out evenly on the second layer. By now, you should have two layers of dough and two layers of chocolate.
- Repeat the same steps with the last chilled dough portion. Place it on a large piece of lightly floured parchment paper. Repeat the same steps of rolling it out about 1/3" thick. Carefully transfer the rolled dough on top of the 2nd layer with the chocolate crumbles. Lastly, taking the remaining chocolate crumbles, spread them out evenly over the top of the 3rd layer of dough.
- Taking your rolling pin, lightly roll the three layers out a bit more until about ½" thick.
- Begin cutting out 2"-2 ½" cookies with a circular cookie cutter and transfer to the prepared baking sheets. Combine and roll out the remaining cookie dough and continue to cut out cookies until the dough is used up.
- Using a pastry brush, lightly brush the tops of the cookies with the whipped egg.
- Bake for 11-12 minutes.

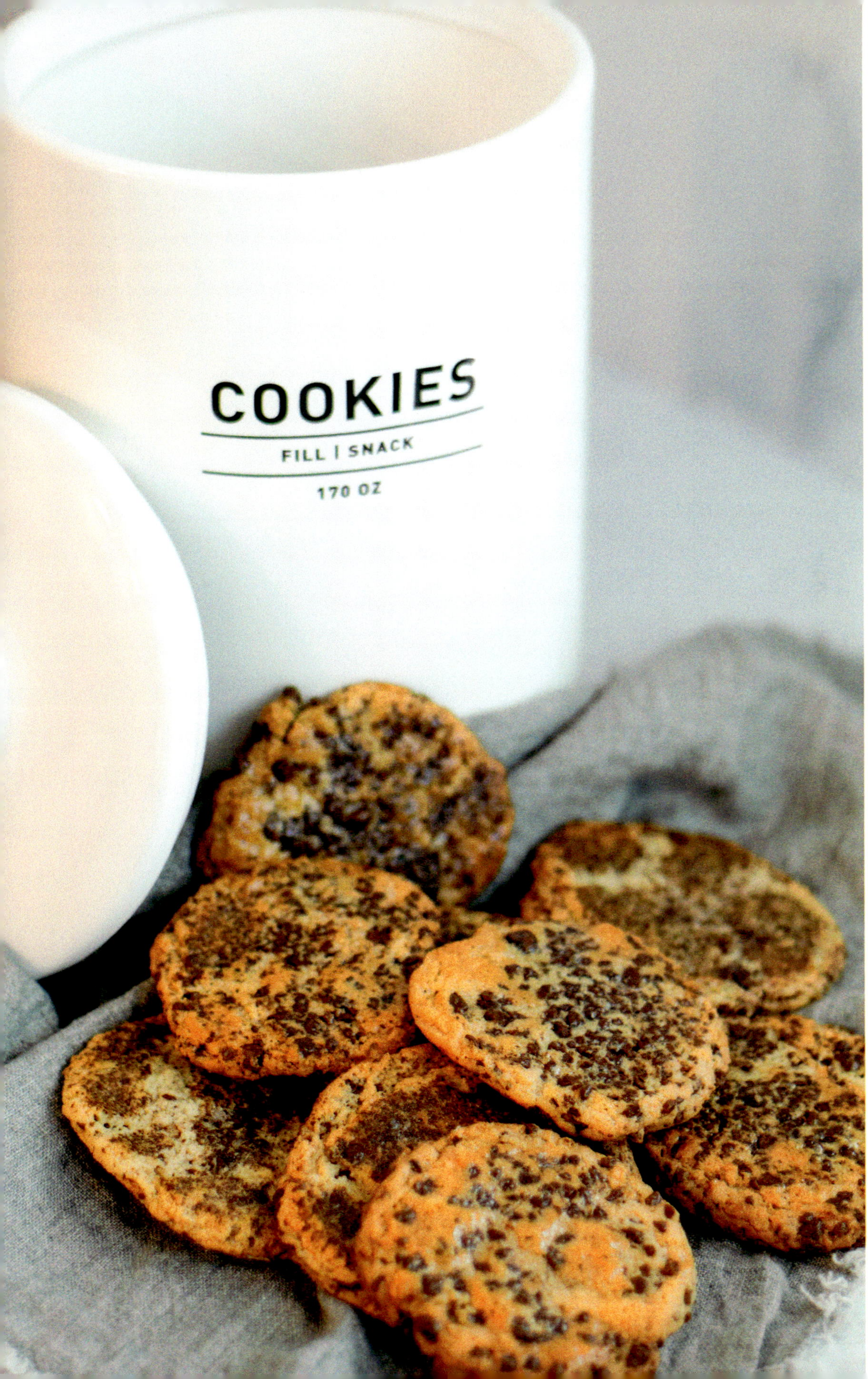

Nut Free

Soy Free

The OG Gingerbread Snickerdoodle Cookies

The OG, the original, the cookie that perhaps started it all. We've called them OSG cookies in the past. These were the very first cookies I ever made for Justin back when we were still dating. I remember baking these cookies in his apartment, not even having proper mixing bowls or a stand mixer. Instead, I used a smoothie blender to cream the butter and sugar together. I still remember how much he loved these cookies the very first time I ever made them. He raved about them for weeks, even had me make them for his parents. Perhaps these cookies were the reason we got married. Maybe these cookies got me started in the kitchen all those years ago. They're simple to make, soft and gooey to bite, they're sweet with a hint of spice, and they pair perfectly with a cold glass of milk.

PREP TIME: 15 minutes

COOK TIME: 10-12 minutes

YIELDS: 19-20 cookies

Ingredients:

¾ cup butter, softened

1 cup granulated sugar

1 large egg

¼ cup pure maple syrup

2 ¼ cup all purpose flour

2 tsp ground ginger

¾ tsp ground cinnamon

½ tsp ground cloves

1 tsp baking soda

Pinch of salt

⅓ cup granulated sugar for rolling cookies

Directions:

- Preheat the oven to 350 degrees Fahrenheit. Prepare 2 baking sheets with parchment paper.
- In a large mixing bowl, cream together the butter and sugar until light and fluffy (about 2-3 minutes). Add the egg and maple syrup and mix until combined.
- In a separate mixing bowl, whisk together the flour, ginger, cinnamon, cloves, baking soda, and salt.
- Combine the flour mixture with the wet ingredients and mix until well combined.
- In a separate small bowl, pour the additional ⅓ cup sugar.
- Roll the cookie dough into 1-1 ½ inch balls. Continue to roll the cookie balls in the sugar to cover well and place on the prepared baking sheets.
- Bake for 10-12 minutes. If you prefer soft, gooey snickerdoodle cookies, pull them out at 10 minutes and let them set.

Tip:

Store in an airtight container for up to 1 week.

☆☆☆☆☆

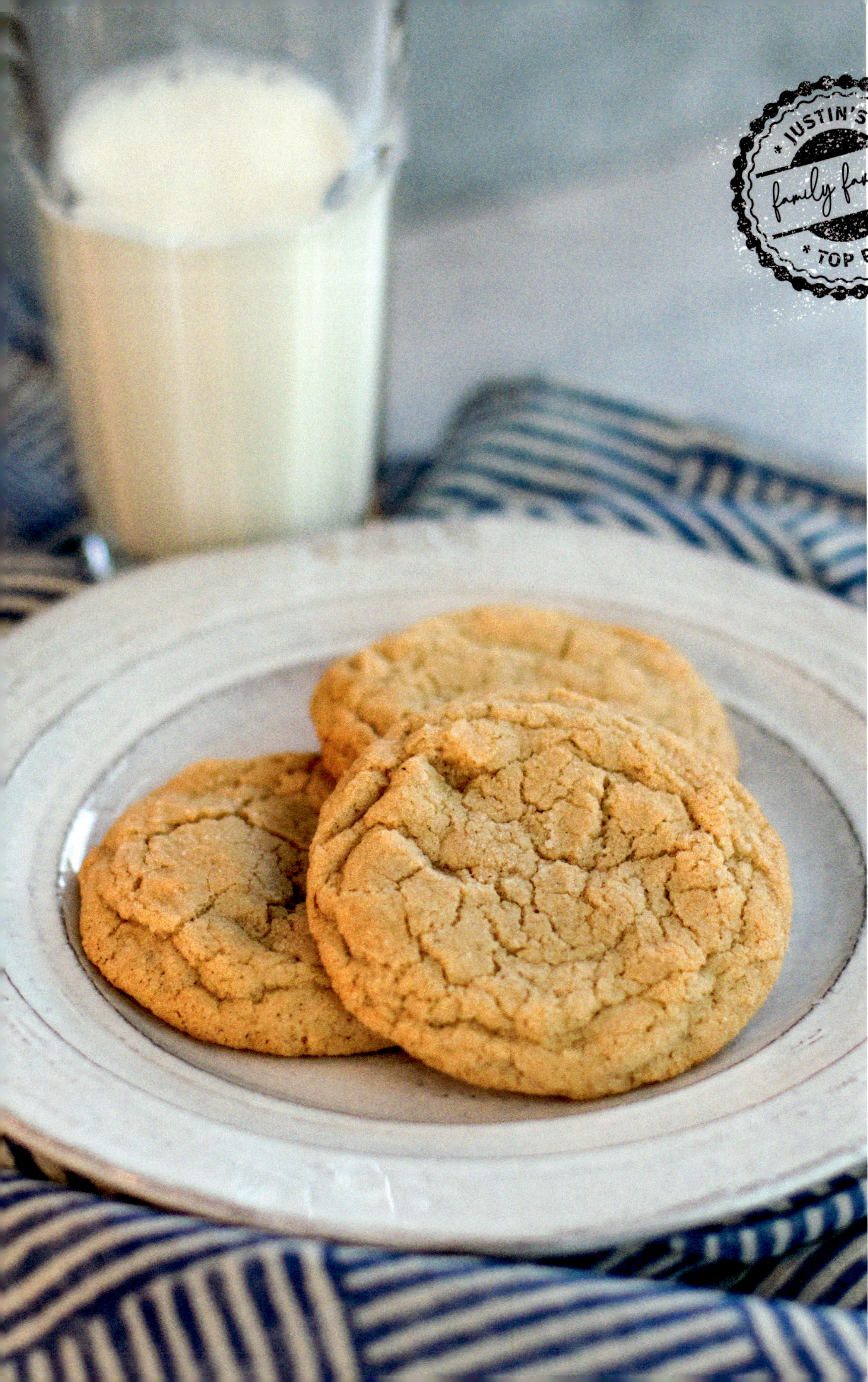

Nut Free

Soy Free

Simple Christmas Gingerbread Cookies

Our first Christmas with Emmie, we were only three months into our parenting journey. Those first three stressful months seemed to fly by; there was so much to do and so much to keep up with. When the Christmas season came, I was adamant about keeping things simple and pure. From decorations to baking and cooking, my theme was simplicity, which is still something I thrive on today. That year I created this simple gingerbread cookie recipe, and it's turned out to be one of my Christmas traditions to give to others because of how easy yet beautiful they turn out. To me, Christmas time shouldn't be about the glitz and glam that social media makes it out to be. Instead, simplicity throughout the season allows us to really focus on what matters most; our faith, our family, our friends.

PREP TIME: 30 minutes

COOK TIME: 08 minutes

YIELDS: Dependent on cookie cutter sizes (20-30 cookies)

Ingredients:

FOR THE COOKIES

10 tbsp butter, softened

¾ cup packed light brown sugar

⅔ cup pure maple syrup

1 large egg

1 tsp pure vanilla extract

3 ½ cup all purpose flour

1 tbsp ground ginger

1 tbsp ground cinnamon

½ tsp pumpkin pie spice

½ tsp ground cloves

1 tsp baking soda

Pinch of salt

FOR THE ROYAL ICING

1 ½ cup confectioner's sugar

½ tsp pure vanilla extract

1 tsp light corn syrup

2 tbsp water

Small pinch of salt

☆☆☆☆☆

Directions:

- Preheat the oven to 350 degrees Fahrenheit. Prepare 2 baking sheets with parchment paper.
- Using an electric mixer and large mixing bowl, cream together the softened butter and brown sugar on medium speed until whipped together. Add the maple syrup and continue to mix together.
- Next, add the egg and the vanilla extract and continue to mix on medium speed until combined.
- In a smaller mixing bowl, combine the flour, ginger, cinnamon, pumpkin pie spice, cloves, baking soda, and salt. Slowly add the dry ingredients to the electric mixer and mix on medium speed until completely combined. You may need to stop the mixer a few times and scrape down the sides.
- Using your hands, separate the dough into two portions and continue to knead each portion until dough is formed into a ball shape.
- On a lightly floured surface, roll the dough out (using flour on the rolling pin as well) until the dough is about 1/3 inch thick. Using cookie cutters of your choice, begin cutting out shapes and placing them on a prepared cookie sheet. Continue to reuse and roll out the scraps until the dough is completely used up. Continue with the second dough ball.
- Bake for 8 minutes or until golden brown and desired cookie softness is achieved.
- While the cookies are baking, begin making the royal icing.

FOR THE ICING

- In an electric mixer and large mixing bowl, combine the confectioner's sugar, vanilla, corn syrup, water, and salt together. Mix until a smooth consistency is formed.
- If the icing is too thick, simply add more water ½ tsp at a time. Careful not to add too much, as the icing should not be drippy.
- Once the cookies are cooled, you can begin decorating the cookies.

Tips:

Cookies can be stored in an airtight container at room temperature for up to 7 days.

Cookie dough can be chilled prior to use for up to 5 days or kept frozen until needed.

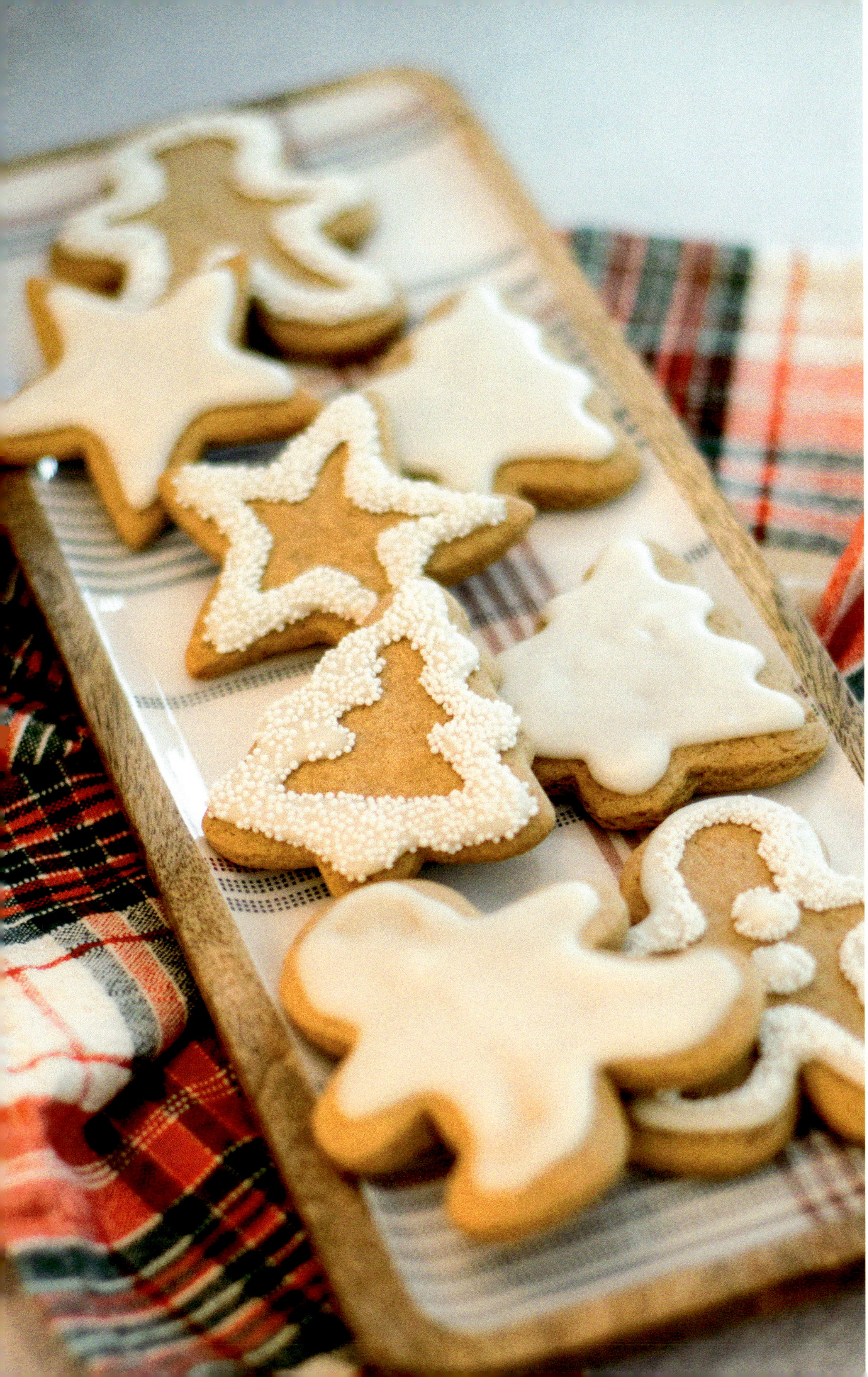

Nut Free

Soy Free

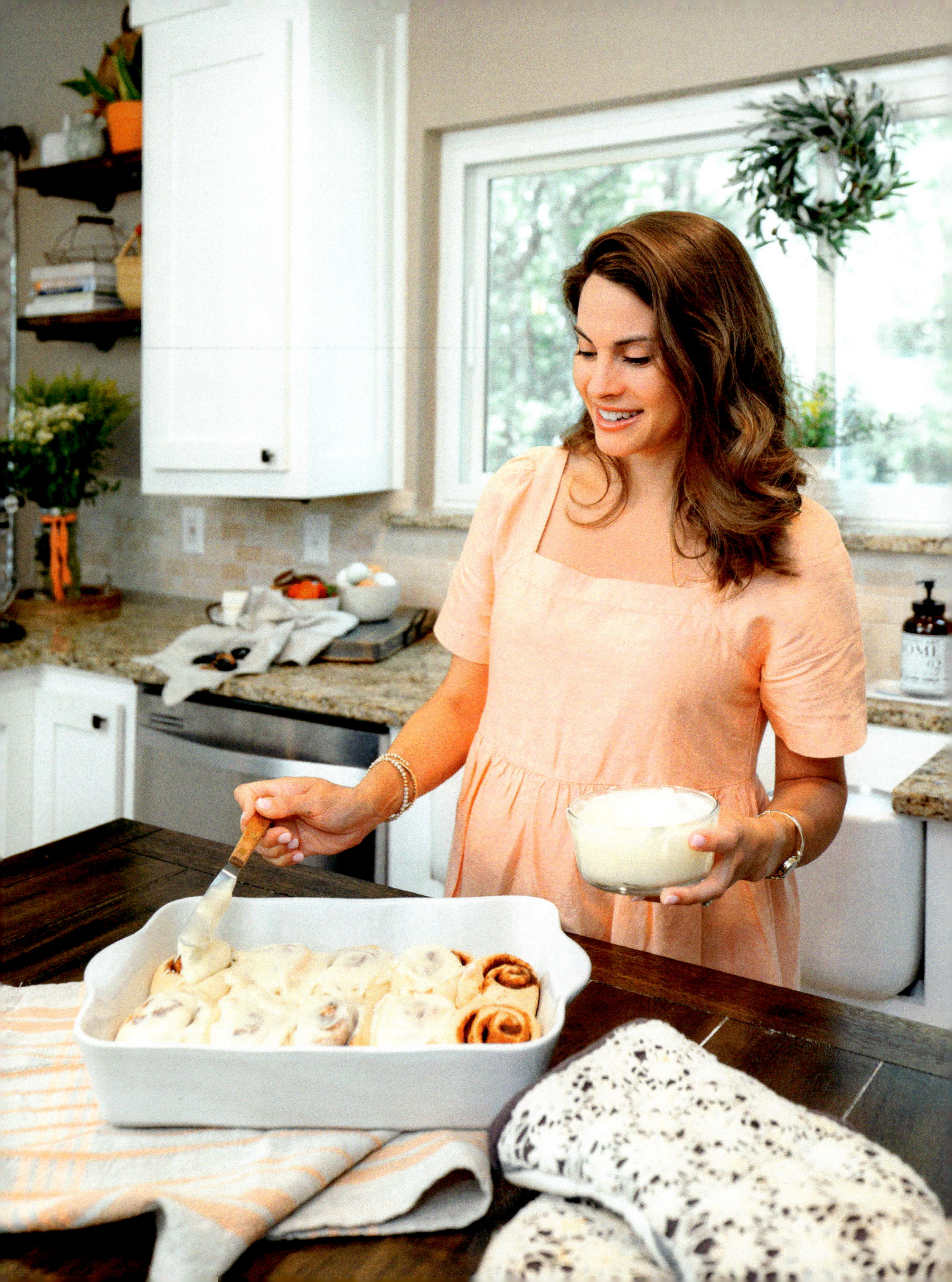

Can't miss these other Sweet Treats

- Gooey Toffee Walnut Blondies
- 10 - Minute Simple Brownies
- Sweet Summer Blackberry Crumble
- Mother's Day Lemon Scones *(Mimi's Pick)*
- AVO Little Chocolate Cake
- Almond Butter Nutty Chow
- No Bake Chocolate Covered Pretzel Bars
- Cranberry Orange Breakfast Muffins *(Tata's Pick)*
- Bacon Breakfast Scones with Maple Glaze
- Pumpkin Pecan Quick Bread
- Sweet & Salty Candied Pecans
- My Infamous Traditional Cinnamon Rolls
- Life's Peachy & Crisp
- Simple Strawberry Rhubarb Jam

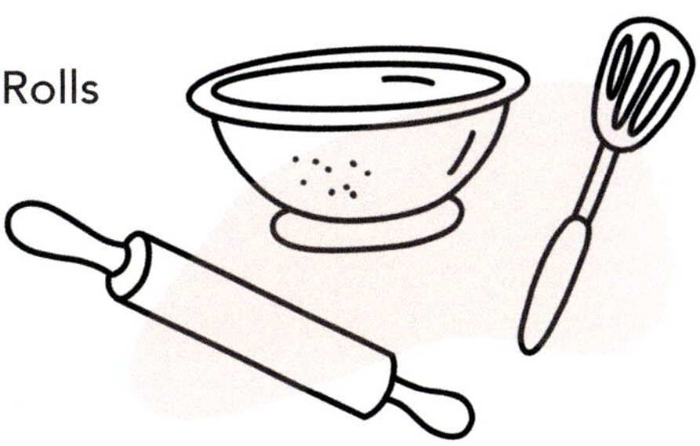

Although this book is primarily a cookie cookbook, I can't help but love this section the most. Maybe it's because the recipes in this section are so incredibly different, yet they all hold a special place in my heart (and tummy).

Most of these recipes have been in the making many years. I've updated and adapted them as the years have progressed and my baking experience has increased. Like the previous section of our family's tried and true cookie favorites, these are among my family's favorite non-cookie desserts. Each of these recipes tell a different story, remind me of a specific time, and I am excited to share these sweet, simple moments with you.

My only suggestion, don't put this book down until you've tried my *traditional cinnamon rolls.*

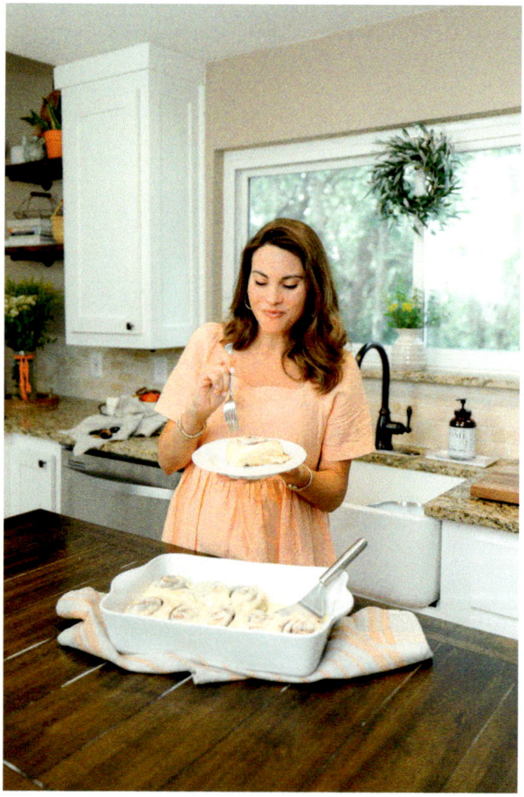

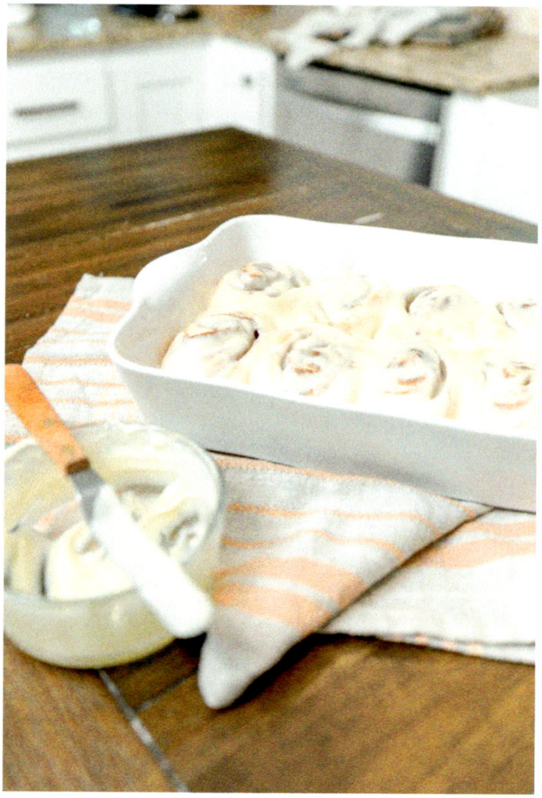

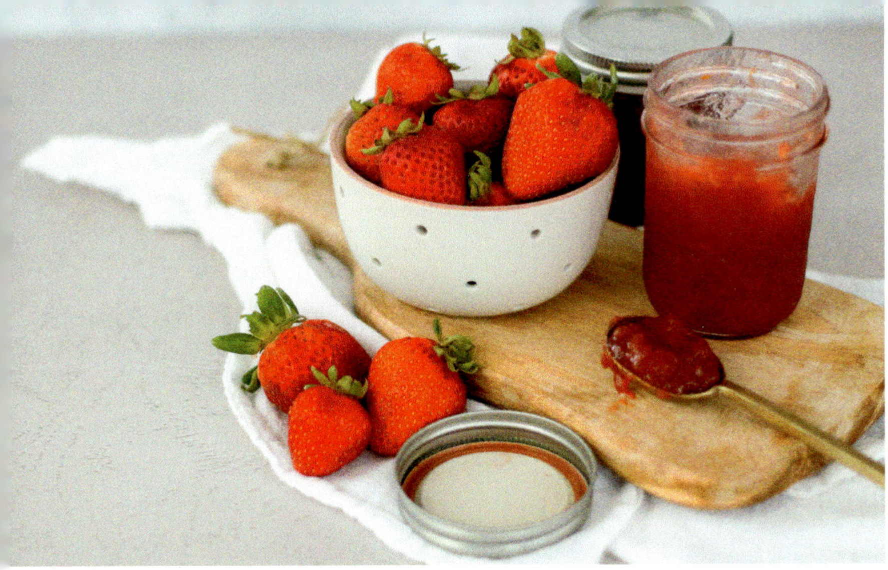

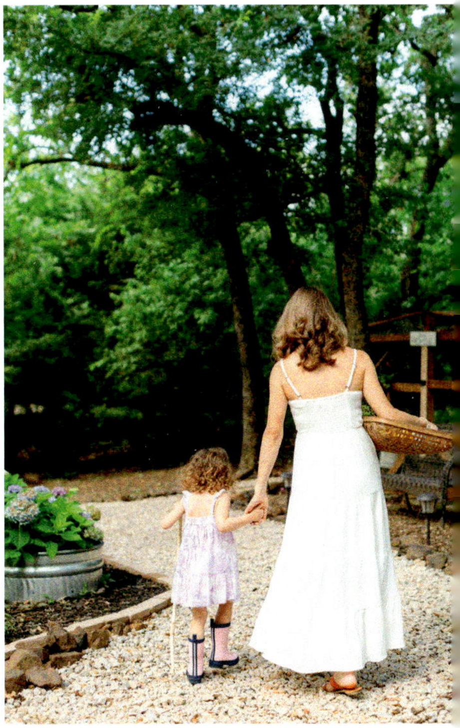

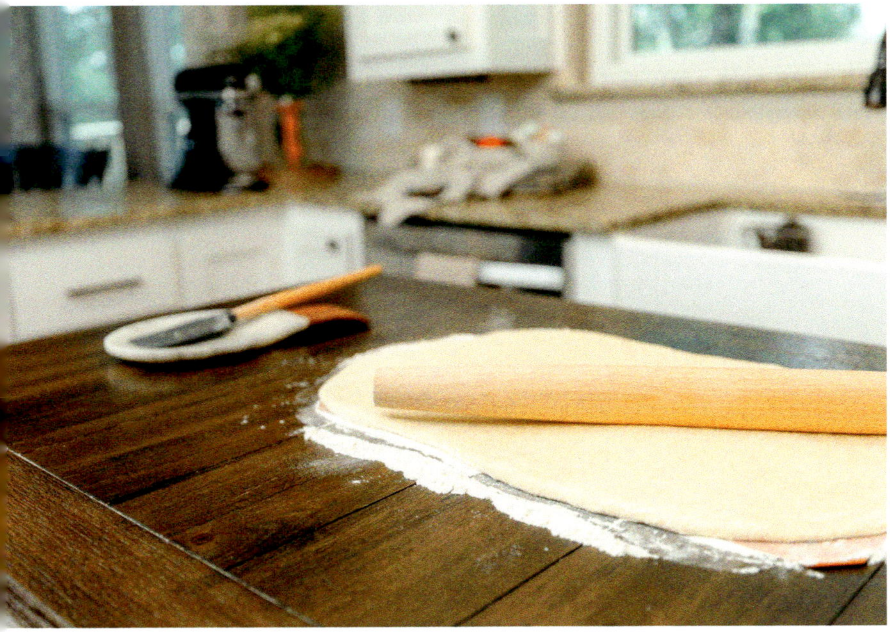

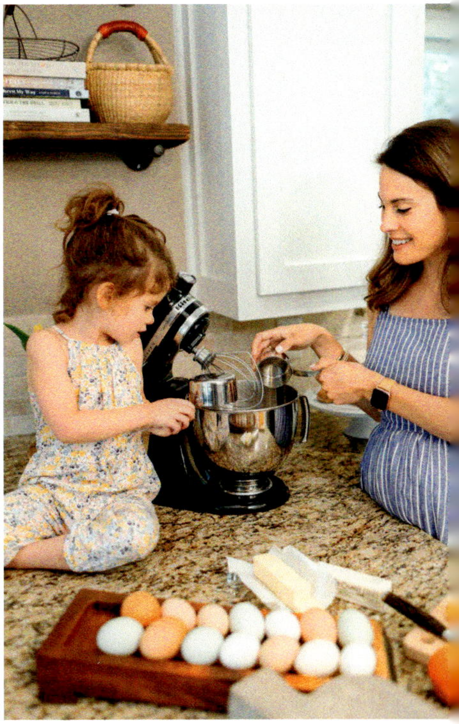

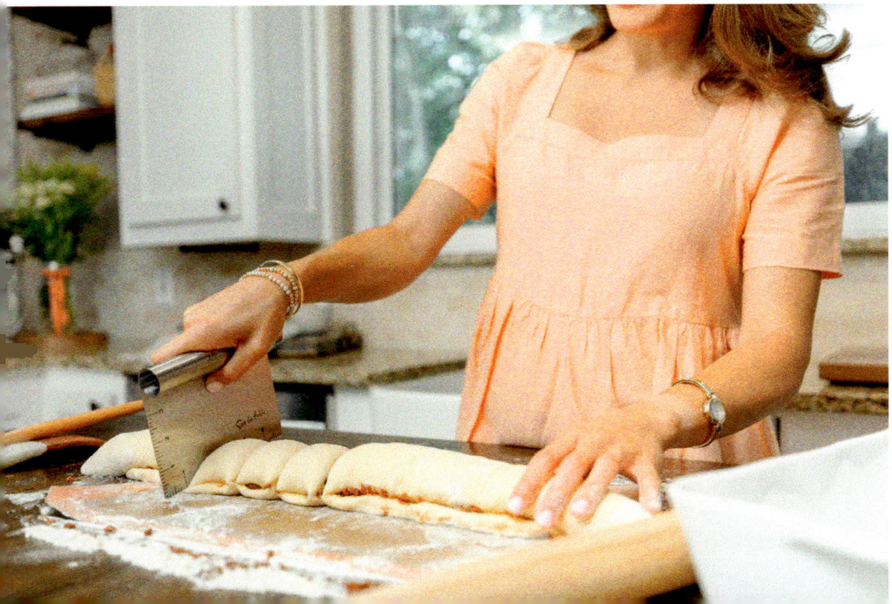

Gooey Toffee Walnut Blondies

If it wasn't for my mother-in-law, I don't think I would have ever known about toffee and the possibilities for dessert. So when I said I wanted to create a blondie recipe for this book, I asked my family if I should include toffee or butterscotch, and the answer was unanimous - toffee was the clear-cut winner. I can now confidently say they chose rightly. Furthermore, I also wanted to include a blondie recipe for those of you who don't indulge in chocolate like Justin. My older brother and I would rather have a warm gooey blondie than a decadent brownie any day. You might call us crazy or rare and unique, but we all have our preferences, and these, my friend, have made the list for my next backyard BBQ dinner instead of traditional brownies. Mindblown? Try them out for yourself and see what we're talking about.

PREP TIME: 15 minutes

COOK TIME: 30 minutes

YIELDS: 12 cookie bars

Ingredients:

1 cup all purpose flour

Pinch of salt

1 tsp baking powder

½ cup butter, melted

1 cup packed light brown sugar

1 large egg + 1 large egg yolk, room temperature

1 tsp pure vanilla extract

½ cup chopped walnuts

1/3 cup toffee bits
(such as Heath English Toffee Bits)

Directions:

- Preheat the oven to 350 degrees Fahrenheit. Prepare an 8x8 inch glass pan with butter or cooking spray (such as avocado oil)
- In a small mixing bowl, combine the flour, salt, and baking powder, set aside.
- In a large mixing bowl, whisk together the melted butter and brown sugar until well combined. Add the eggs and vanilla extract and continue to whisk until smooth.
- Add the dry ingredients to the butter mixture and whisk again until smooth.
- Using a spatula, fold in the walnuts and toffee bits.
- Pour the batter into the prepared baking pan. Using the spatula, push the batter to the corners of the pan and level out until smooth.
- Bake for 20 minutes then place aluminum foil on top to prevent too much browning. Continue to bake for another 10 minutes.
- Using a toothpick, submerge into the center and pull it out. If it remains clean, the blondies are done, if the toothpick comes out gooey, continue to bake until the toothpick comes out clean (about 1-3 minutes).

Tip:

Store in an airtight container for up to 7 days.

☆☆☆☆☆

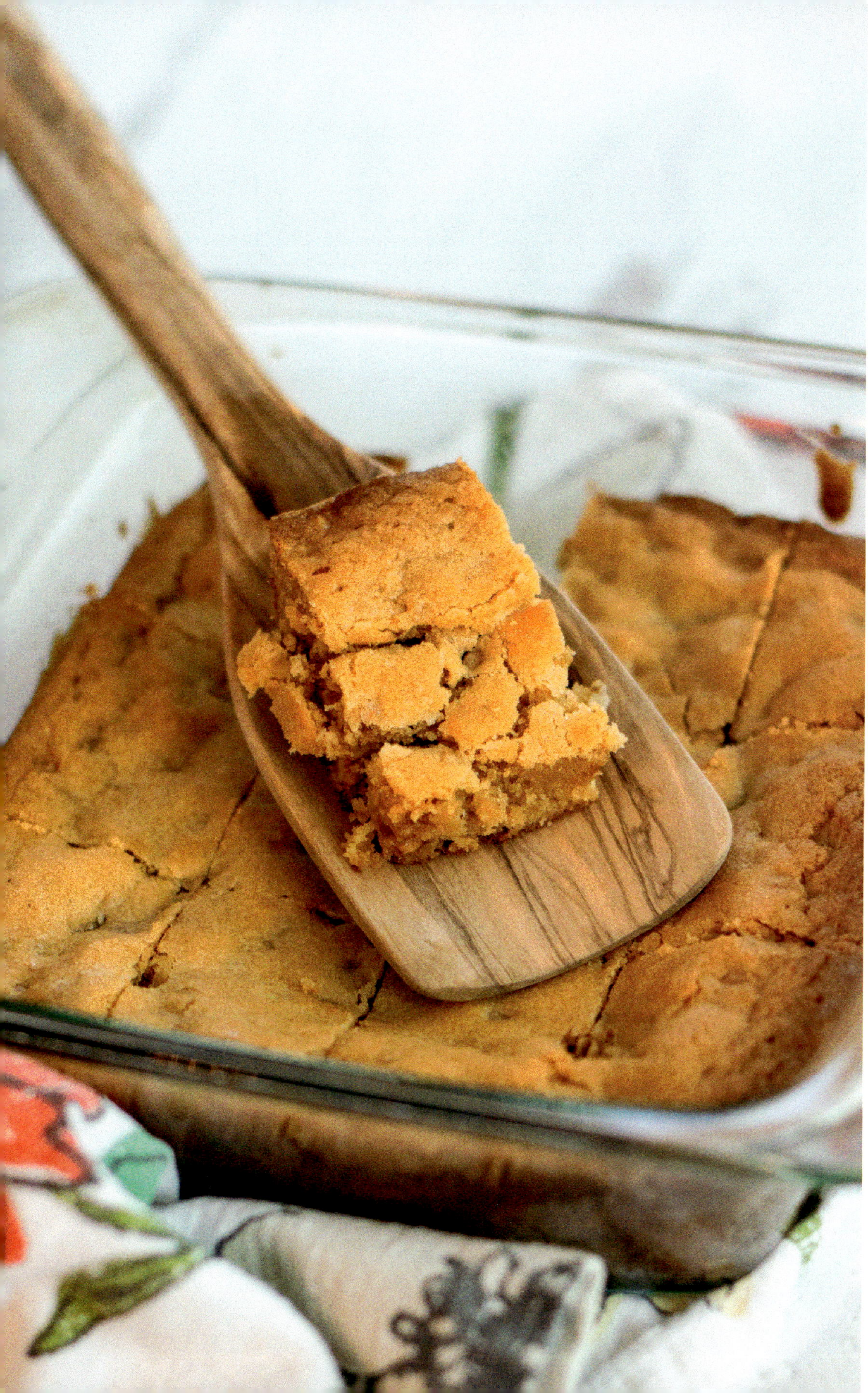

10-Minute Simple Brownies

These brownies have changed my baking game. Seriously. This recipe is the base for so many of my chocolate-themed cookies in this book because the texture, taste, and simplicity make them so perfect for any occasion. Need a last-minute dessert to bring to the pool party? This is it. Need a last-minute dessert for a potluck, wine night, picnic, or holiday meal? This is it. Brownies are usually a safe crowd favorite, and these pair perfectly with just about anything. Think warm brownie with a scoop of cold vanilla ice cream, a drizzle of rich chocolate ganache, or even a scoop of homemade whipped cream.

PREP TIME: 10 minutes

COOK TIME: 30-35 minutes

YIELDS: 12 brownie squares

Ingredients:

10 tbsp butter, softened

1 cup granulated sugar

2 large eggs, room temperature

1 tsp pure vanilla extract

½ cup 100% naturally unsweetened cocoa powder

½ cup all purpose flour

Pinch of salt

½ cup chopped walnuts

Optional Topping:
Himalayan salt

Directions:

- Preheat the oven to 325 degrees Fahrenheit. Prepare an 8" or 9" square baking dish with parchment paper and or avocado cooking spray to prevent the brownies from sticking.
- In a large mixing bowl, cream together the butter and sugar until light and fluffy (about 2-3 minutes). Add the eggs and vanilla and mix until combined.
- In a separate mixing bowl, whisk together the cocoa powder, flour, and salt.
- Combine the flour mixture with the wet ingredients and mix until well combined.
- Fold in the walnuts.
- Pour the batter into the prepared square baking dish. Using a rubber spatula, push the batter into the corners and smooth it out until leveled.
- Bake for 30-35 minutes or until a toothpick inserted into the middle of the brownies comes out clean.
- After taking the brownies out of the oven, top with optional pink Himalayan salt.
- Let cool completely before cutting into squares.

Tips:

Can be stored at room temperature with aluminum foil or plastic wrap to cover the top.

Perfect for serving with vanilla ice cream or a cold glass of milk.

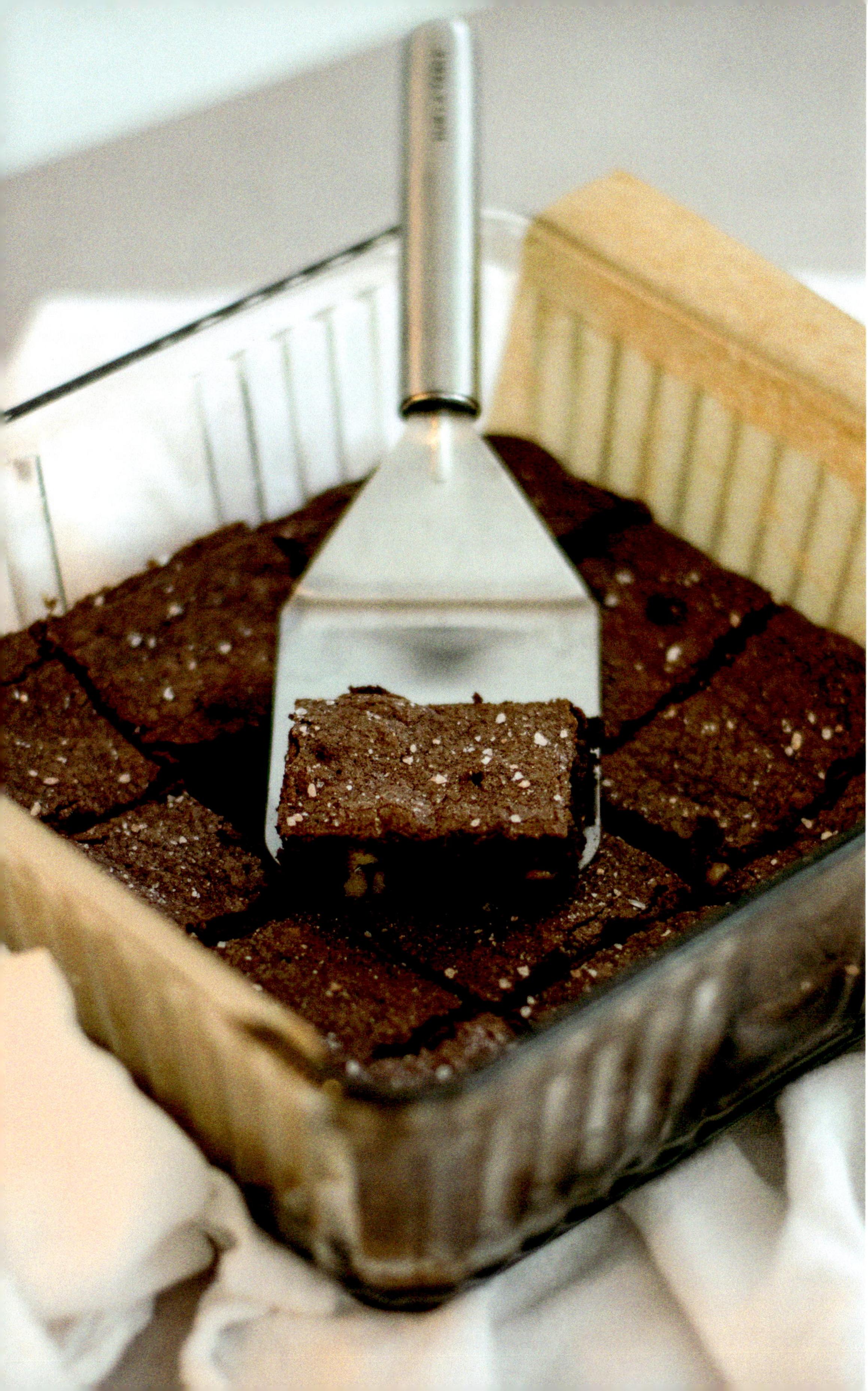

Soy Free

Sweet Summer Blackberry Crumble

Few things in life are sweeter than fresh-picked berries in the summer. From strawberries to raspberries to blackberries, I find myself running back to the grocery store or local farmer's market every time I run low on berry inventory. I must have passed my love for fruit on to Emmie because she gobbles them up just as fast as I do. One reason I love making this crumble in the summertime is the accessibility to fresh blackberries. They make the whole crumble taste so light and fresh, you might even find yourself serving it up for breakfast. You can still use frozen blackberries to create a delicious treat during the off-season, making this recipe enjoyable year-round.

PREP TIME: 20 minutes

COOK TIME: 30-35 minutes

YIELDS: 9 servings

Ingredients:

4 cups rinsed, fresh blackberries (or frozen when not in season)

½ cup granulated sugar

1 medium-sized lemon, zested

1 tsp ground cinnamon

¾ cup all purpose flour

¼ cup granulated sugar

6 tbsp cold salted butter, cut into tbsp pats

½ cup old fashioned rolled oats

1 tbsp pure maple syrup

¼ cup sliced almonds

Directions:

- Preheat the oven to 375 degrees Fahrenheit and prepare the bottom and sides of an 8x8 or 9x9 inch square glass baking dish.
- In a mixing bowl, combine the blackberries, sugar, lemon zest, and cinnamon together. Mix together well and pour into the prepared baking dish.
- In a separate clean mixing bowl, whisk the flour and sugar together. Add the butter and cut into the flour using a pastry cutter or your hands.
- In the same mixing bowl, add the rolled oats, maple syrup, and sliced almonds, mix together well. Layer the flour mixture on top of the blackberries, spreading it out evenly to the corners and sides.
- Bake at 375 degrees for 30-35 minutes or until the rolled oats begin to turn golden and the fruit is slightly bubbling. Let cool on a cooling rack before serving.

Tips:

Can be stored at room temperature or in the refrigerator with aluminum foil or plastic wrap to cover the top.

Perfect to serve with vanilla ice cream or a cold glass of milk.

☆☆☆☆☆

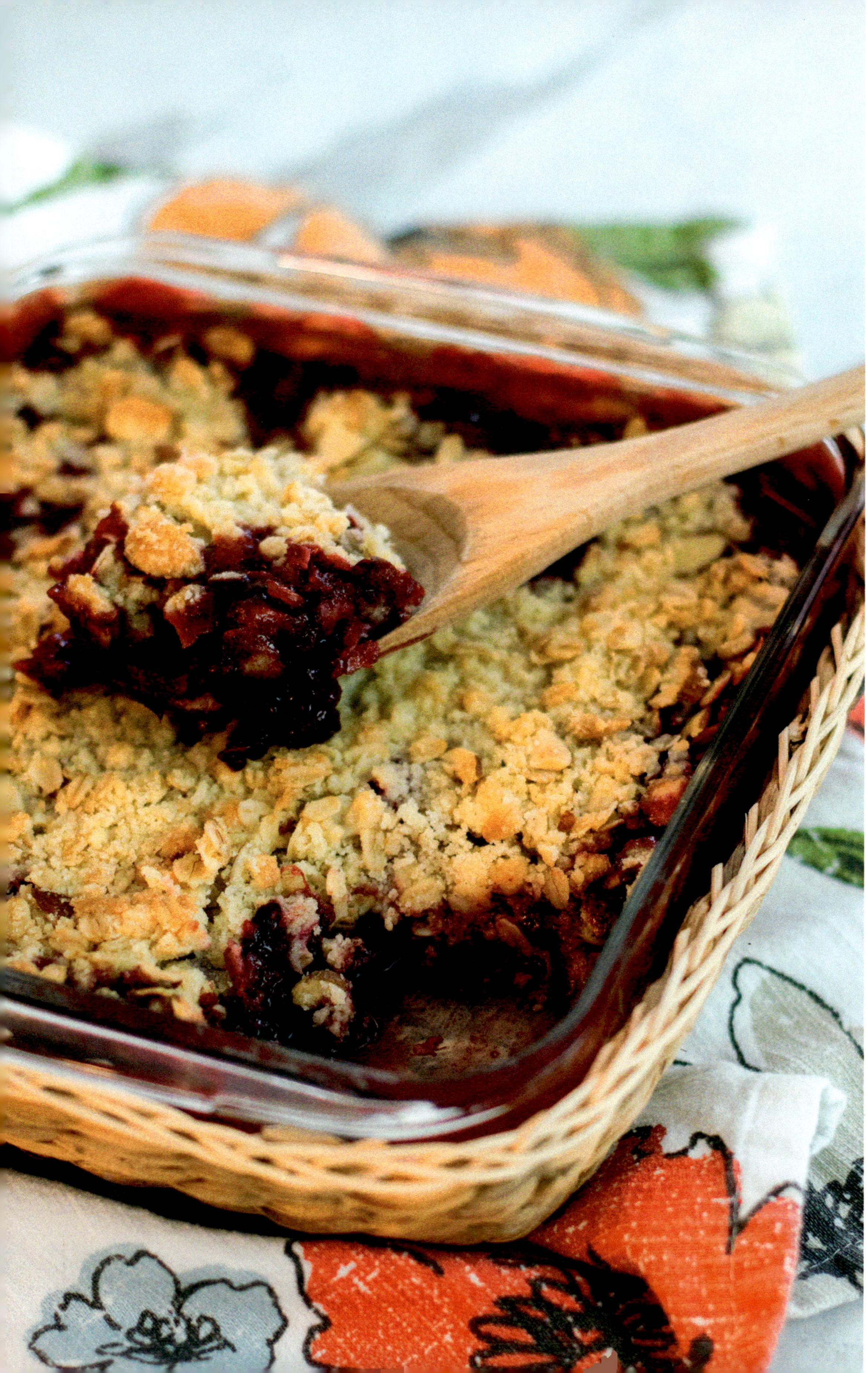

Egg Free

Soy Free

Mother's Day Lemon Scones

My Mother-in-law, Mimi, loves lemon scones. For mother's day one year, I made fresh lemon scones to help celebrate our day together. Now, whenever I make a fresh batch, I know I'll be in trouble if I don't share at least a few with her. Her favorite way to enjoy them is over a cup of coffee in the morning. For me, I enjoy them any time of the day as a sweet pick-me-up and a way to unwind from the day's craziness.

Since creating this recipe a few years ago, I have adapted and changed it. This recipe was first featured in my "Spring to Summer" recipe ebook; however, I have made one simple change that has drastically changed its texture. Make sure to use heavy whipping cream when baking these scones instead of half-and-half. The extra fat content helps bind the scones together while baking for a soft yet delicate crumbly texture. These scones may be a tad time & labor-intensive, but they sure make for a wonderful gift.

PREP TIME: 35 minutes

COOK TIME: 18-20 minutes

YIELDS: 16 scones

Ingredients:

FOR THE SCONES

2 ¾ cup all purpose flour

1 tsp baking powder

1 cup packed confectioner's sugar

1/3 cup granulated sugar

pinch of salt

Zest from 2 large lemons

Juice from 1 large lemon

½ cup heavy whipping cream

½ tsp pure vanilla extract

½ cup cold butter, cut into tbsp pieces

FOR THE GLAZE

1 cup confectioner's sugar

2 tbsp pure maple syrup

½ tsp pure vanilla extract

Zest from 1 large lemon

Juice of 1 large lemon

☆☆☆☆☆

Directions:

FOR THE SCONES

- Preheat the oven to 375 degrees Fahrenheit and prepare a large baking sheet with parchment paper.
- In a large mixing bowl, combine the flour, baking powder, confectioner's sugar, granulated sugar, salt, and lemon zest. Whisk together until well incorporated, set aside.
- In a smaller mixing bowl, whisk together the heavy cream, lemon juice, and vanilla extract. Set aside.
- Using a pastry cutter, begin cutting the chilled butter into the flour mixture until the butter pieces resemble tiny balls. You can also use a food processor to save time and arm strength, but it is not necessary.
- Pour the liquid heavy cream mixture into the flour. Using a rubber spatula or your hands, begin mixing the dough. The dough will be incredibly hard to incorporate; you might think it's too dry and crumbly but continue to work with it. It will eventually mold together perfectly.
- Place the dough on a lightly floured work surface. Using a rolling pin and pastry scarper, begin to shape into a rectangle (about ½" thick). Once the dough is shaped and rolled evenly, using the pastry scraper, slice into 16 mini triangles.
- Place the triangles on the prepared baking sheet as you would cookies and cook for 18-20 minutes or until slightly golden brown on the edges.

FOR THE GLAZE

- While the scones are baking, in a small bowl, whisk together the remaining ingredients until smooth (confectioners sugar, maple syrup, vanilla, lemon zest, and lemon juice). After the scones are done baking and cooled, brush 2-3 coats of the glaze on top, allowing to set between coats.

Tip:

Store in an airtight container either in the fridge or countertop for up to 5-6 days.

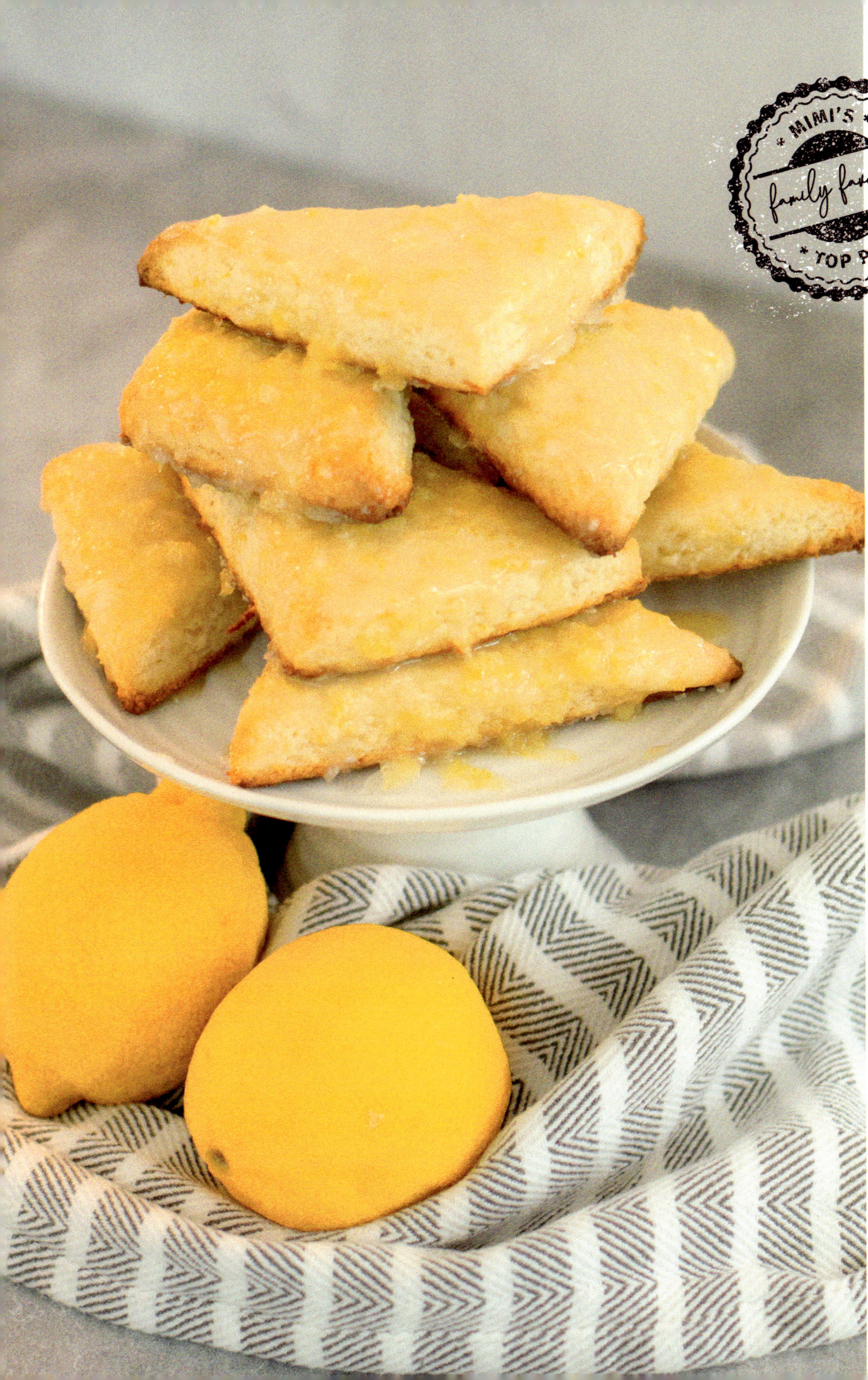

Nut Free

Egg Free

Soy Free

AVO Little Chocolate Cake

These days, the trend of putting avocado in chocolate cake isn't anything new, but these little cakes might make you think about dessert in a different light. Full of healthy fats without all the butter, these little bundt cakes will have you reaching for more without hesitation. Although slightly dense, the avocado creates a moist texture that more than makes up for the missing creamed butter. This is one of my favorite recipes to make around Valentine's Day because of the simplicity and presentation of fresh-cut strawberries on top of whipped cream and chocolate cake.

PREP TIME: 25 minutes

COOK TIME: 18 minutes

YIELDS: 6 mini bundt cakes

Ingredients:

FOR THE CAKE

3 large eggs

1 ½ cup granulated sugar

1 medium-sized avocado, mashed

2 tsp pure vanilla extract

¾ cup all purpose flour

¾ cup 100% naturally unsweetened cocoa powder

1 tsp baking powder

Pinch of salt

FOR THE WHIPPED CREAM

1 ½ cup heavy whipping cream

3 tbsp granulated sugar

1 tsp pure vanilla extract

Directions:

- Preheat the oven to 350 degrees Fahrenheit. Prepare a baking pan with 6 mini bundt cake molds with cooking spray (such as avocado oil) to prevent sticking.
- Using an electric mixer, mix together the eggs, granulated sugar, and mashed avocado on medium speed until most of the avocado is broken down into tiny pieces. Add the vanilla extract and continue to mix until combined.
- In a small mixing bowl, whisk together the flour, cocoa powder, baking powder, and salt. Add the dry ingredients to the wet ingredients and mix until just combined. You may need to stop the mixer and scrape down the sides of the bowl as needed.
- Spoon the prepared batter into each mini bundt cake mold about ¾ full.
- Bake for 18 minutes. When done baking, use a toothpick to poke the center of a single bundt cake to determine if it is ready (the toothpick should come out clean).
- Let the cakes cool completely before taking out the molds. When done cooling, flip the baking pan upside down on a wire cooling rack to allow for the cakes to drop out of the molds (I usually have to loosen the molds with a small rubber spatula first).
- While the bundt cakes are cooling, begin making the whipped cream. Using an electric mixer, cream together the heavy whipping cream, sugar, and vanilla until soft peaks begin to form and desired texture is achieved (about 5-10 minutes on medium-high speed).
- Top the cooled cakes with a spoonful of fresh whipped cream and optional fruit topping such as cut strawberries.

Tips:

Store cakes and whipped cream in the fridge for up to 5 days.

Cakes are best served warm with chilled whipped cream and fruit topping of choice.

Dairy-free Coconut cream frosting can be used instead of whipped cream if a dairy allergy is present. See Pumpkin Spice Snickerdoodle for recipe reference.

☆☆☆☆☆

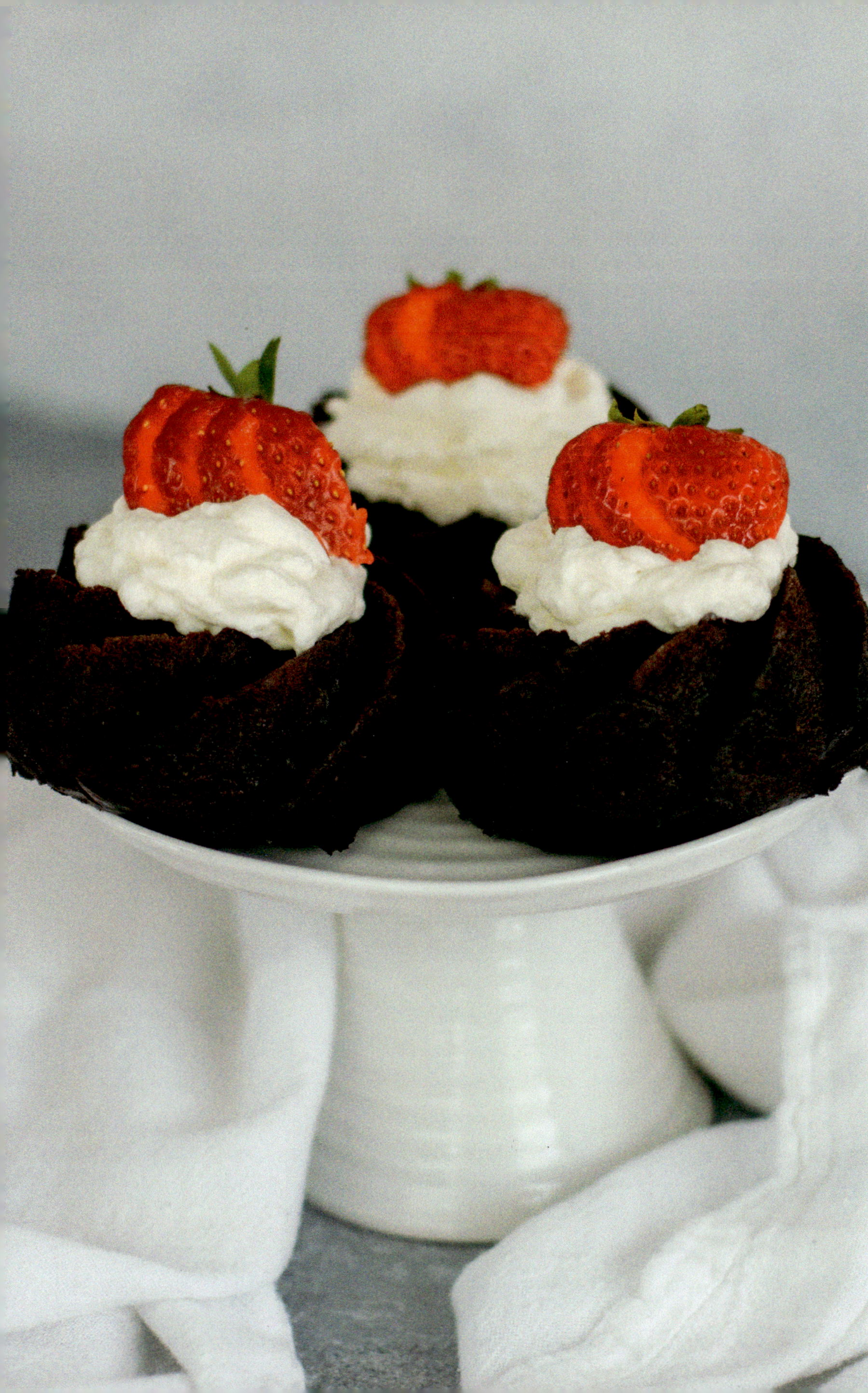

Dairy Free (without the whipped cream)

Nut Free

Soy Free

Almond Butter Nutty Chow

In case you've never had the wonderful opportunity of making Puppy Chow throughout your childhood, it's a fairly easy (no-bake yet highly addictive) treat to put together. I distinctly remember making puppy chow throughout my high school career, bringing it to school on football game days to share with the rest of my dance squad and football players. So I put this recipe together to create a healthy(er) version of the sugary treat. This version contains dried fruit, three different varieties of nuts, and uses coconut oil instead of butter. But who's counting? This candy dish is perfect for bringing to a Halloween party for its bright and bold orange colors. It's also easy to bag up and hand out to kids who visit your house or even munch on for a dessert.

PREP TIME: 15 minutes

COOK TIME: No Bake

YIELDS: ~15 cups of chow

Ingredients:

12 oz box original Rice Chex™

1 cup walnuts, chopped

1 cup cashews, chopped

1 cup macadamia nuts, halved

¾ cup creamy style almond butter

1 cup dark chocolate chips

2 tbsp coconut oil

1 tsp pure vanilla extract

2 cup confectioner's sugar

¾ cup golden raisins

¾ cup dried apricots, chopped

Directions:

- In a large mixing bowl, combine the Rice Chex™, walnuts, cashews, and macadamia nuts together. Set aside for later use.
- In a microwavable glass bowl, combine the almond butter, chocolate chips, and coconut oil together. Heat in the microwave for 1 minute. Using a rubber spatula, stir together and place back in the microwave for another 30 seconds.
- Add the vanilla and stir well until smoothly incorporated.
- Pour the melted chocolate mixture on the Chex™ mixture and gently mix until evenly coated. Transfer the Chex™ into a large Tupperware container with a lid.
- Add the confectioner's sugar, place the lid on top and shake the container until the Chex™ are evenly coated.
- Lastly, top with golden raisins and dried apricots.

Tips:

It can be stored at room temperature or in the refrigerator with aluminum foil or plastic wrap to cover the top.

Additional toppings can include pretzels, mini chocolate chips, m&m's™, etc.

☆☆☆☆☆

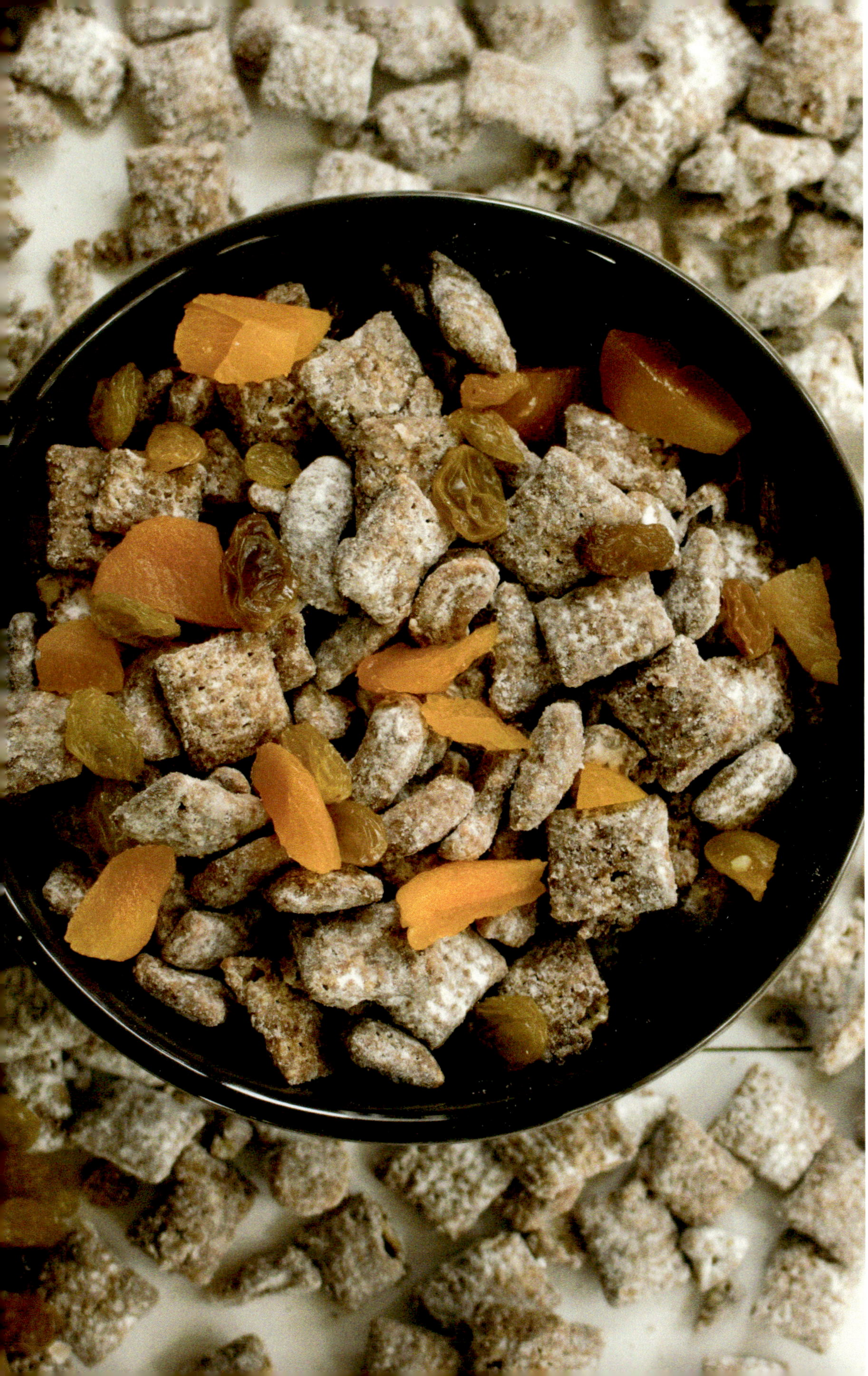

Egg Free

Gluten Free

Dairy Free

Soy Free

No Bake Chocolate Covered Pretzel Bars

Sweet and salty are at it again with these easy pretzel bars. Perfect to take with you or put inside a lunchbox for a midday snack; they are the perfect silencer to that chocolate craving you've been having. With such simple ingredients, you know exactly what you're enjoying instead of questioning that highly processed, self-stable candy bar. Furthermore, you can enjoy these pretzel bars year-round. Because they are no-bake, they become even sweeter in the summertime when the last thing you want to do is turn on your oven for an hour's worth of baking. My trick is putting them in the freezer for when the dog days of summer come. Then I can pull one out and pair it with some ice cream for an added cooling bonus.

PREP TIME: 30 minutes

COOK TIME: No Bake

YIELDS: About 25 square bars

Ingredients:

2 (10 oz) bags of semi-sweet chocolate chips

1 cup coconut milk or heavy whipping cream

1 cup creamy style almond butter or peanut butter

3 cups mini pretzels

Coarse sea salt or pink Himalayan salt

Directions:

- Prepare a baking sheet by covering it with parchment paper.
- Pour one bag of semi-sweet chocolate chips and ½ cup of coconut milk into a microwaveable bowl. Begin melting in the microwave for one minute at a time, stirring occasionally. When melted, mix together well until a smooth consistency is achieved.
- Pour the melted chocolate mixture on the parchment paper and spread it out evenly with a spatula into a rectangular shape. It should be about 12" by 18."
- Place in the refrigerator for about 30-60 minutes to chill. When firm, begin spreading a layer of almond butter over the chocolate.
- Take the mini pretzels and press them gently into the almond butter molding. Place back in the refrigerator to chill.
- Repeat step #2 with the second bag of chocolate and the remaining coconut milk. Evenly spread the melted chocolate over the pretzels. Sprinkle the coarse sea salt over the chocolate and place it back in the refrigerator to chill.
- When the second layer of chocolate is firm, cut into 2" square bars using a sharp knife.

Tip:

Store in an airtight container in the refrigerator for up to 1 week.

☆☆☆☆☆

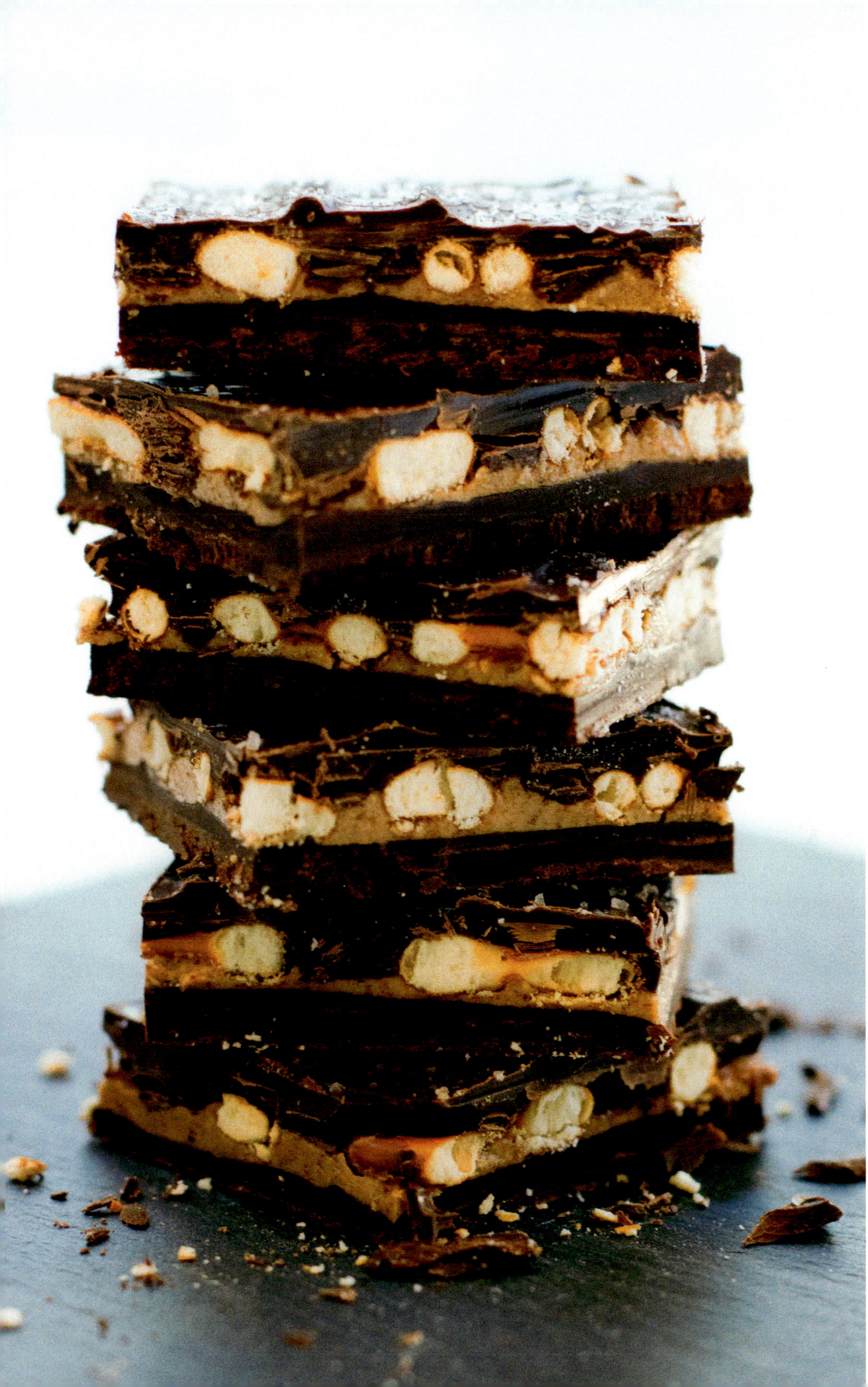

Egg Free

Dairy Free

Soy Free

Cranberry Orange Breakfast Muffins

I'm a big fan of sweet and starchy breakfast items. In fact, it's my weakness. Considering I am a Dietitian and I understand the importance of incorporating healthy fats, protein, and fiber along with those morning carbs, I try to aim for a balanced breakfast every day. These little muffins are the perfect combination of carbohydrates with added fiber (walnuts). However, we enjoy them even more after toasting and smearing them with almond butter to get the added healthy fats. If you're looking for an added boost of protein in the morning, combine a muffin with some scrambled eggs, and you've got yourself a winning combination before heading off to workout, school, or the office.

PREP TIME: 25 minutes

COOK TIME: 20-24 minutes

YIELDS: 12 regular sized muffins

Ingredients:

2 cups all purpose flour

1 tsp baking soda

1 tsp baking powder

Pinch of salt

¾ cup granulated sugar

½ cup unsweetened applesauce

2 large eggs

¼ cup canola or melted coconut oil

1 tsp pure vanilla extract

1 large orange, zested (about 2 tbsp)

1 large orange, juiced (about 4 tbsp)

1 ½ cup whole fresh cranberries

½ cup chopped walnuts

Directions:

- Preheat the oven to 325 degrees Fahrenheit. Prepare a regular-sized, 12-mold muffin tin with cooking spray such as avocado oil.
- In a small mixing bowl, whisk together the flour, baking soda, baking powder, and salt. Set aside for later use.
- In a large-sized mixing bowl, combine the sugar, applesauce, and eggs. Using a whisk, blend the ingredients together well. Once blended, add the oil and vanilla and continue to blend together.
- Slowly pour the dry ingredients into the large mixing bowl and blend together using the whisk. Add the orange zest and juice and blend until well incorporated.
- Using a rubber spatula, fold the cranberries and chopped walnuts into the batter.
- Spoon out the batter into the prepared muffin tin, each mold about ¾ full.
- Place in the oven to bake for 20-24 minutes. Using a toothpick, poke the center of a muffin to determine when done (the toothpick should come out clean). *Can be stored at room temperature or in the refrigerator with aluminum foil or plastic wrap to cover the top.

Tip:

Best served warm with a spoonful of almond butter on top.

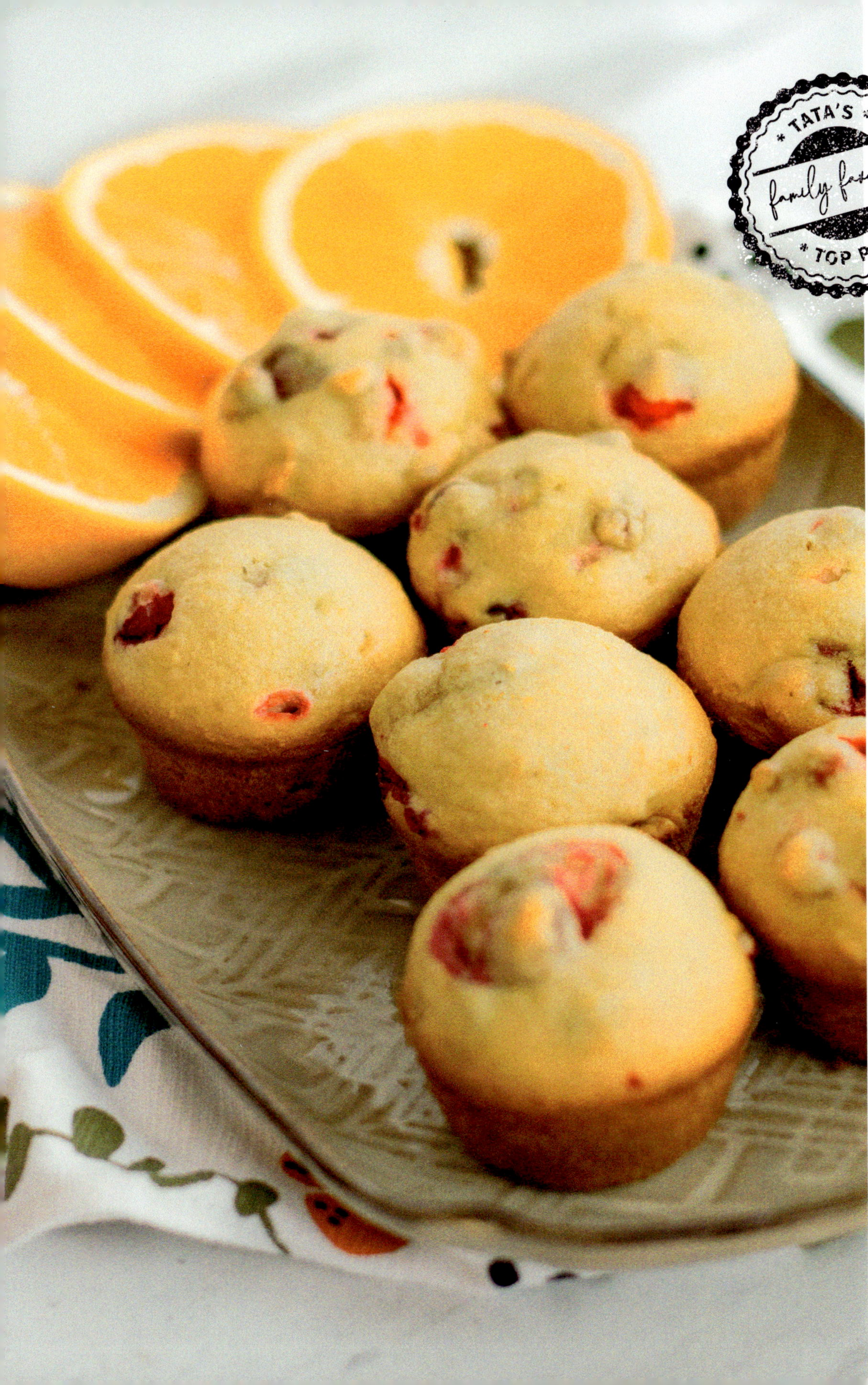

Dairy Free

Soy Free

Bacon Breakfast Scones with Maple Glaze

When I think of a bed and breakfast in the serene Hill Country of Texas, I think of a cozy yet unparalleled breakfast. I think of the fresh-pressed juices, the locally-sourced ingredients, the fresh-out-of-the-oven pastries, and the chef's specialty dishes. I'm a sucker for original and unique creations like those offered in quant bakeries and bed and breakfasts because I feel it makes the food that much more enjoyable to eat. When food has a story behind it, there's life and creativity behind it as well. These creative bacon scones aren't your typical scones found in Starbucks, but to me, that's what makes them even better. Enjoy them for breakfast, as a snack, treat, or dessert- there's no wrong time to enjoy a scone on this level. Inspiration for this recipe came from our favorite Texas Hill Country bed and breakfast, The Sage Hill Inn and Spa on Onion Creek.

PREP TIME: 30 minutes

COOK TIME: 20 minutes

YIELDS: 16 large scones or 32 small scones

Ingredients:

FOR THE DOUGH

2 ¾ cup all purpose flour

1 tsp baking powder

1 tsp baking soda

1 cup packed confectioner's sugar

½ cup granulated sugar

Pinch of salt

½ cup heavy whipping cream

1 tsp pure vanilla extract

1 cup cold butter, cut into tbsp pieces

1 cup chopped cooked bacon

FOR THE GLAZE

3 tbsp butter

½ cup packed light brown sugar

2 tbsp heavy whipping cream

½ cup confectioners sugar

Tip:

Store in an airtight container in the fridge for up to 6 days.

Directions:

- Preheat the oven to 375 degrees Fahrenheit. Prepare 1 baking sheet (if making large scones, 2 baking sheets if making small scones) with parchment paper.
- In an extra-large mixing bowl, whisk together the flour, baking powder, baking soda, confectioner's sugar, granulated sugar, and salt. Set aside.
- In a separate small mixing bowl, whisk together the heavy cream and vanilla extract, set aside.
- Using a pastry cutter, begin cutting the cold butter into the flour mixture until the flour resembles tiny peas and is consistent throughout.
- Pour the heavy cream into the flour mixture. Using a sturdy spatula, begin incorporating the dough together as much as possible. Once the dough gets thick and unable to use the spatula easily, begin using your hands to knead the dough. The dough starts out tough to combine, and you will be tempted to add more liquid; however, it is important to keep kneading the dough as is. Keep shaping until all the flour has been incorporated (it may take about 5-10 minutes of manually kneading). It should come together to form one large, heavy dough ball; if there is dry flour still in the mixing bowl, keep working it. This takes some muscle, but you've got this!
- Fold in the chopped bacon and continue to work with the dough until the bacon is dispersed evenly. However, do not overwork the dough at this point.
- Roll the dough out on a generously floured surface (I prefer to use a slipmat for easier clean up) using a dough scraper, mold, and shape the dough into a rectangle about 3/4 inch thick. (If you don't have a dough scraper, you can use any tool such as a ruler with a straight edge to achieve this).
- To shape the large scone triangles: Slice midway horizontally to create two even long rectangles. Next, slice both rectangles down the middle vertically. Third, slice down the middle of the newly created squares to produce eight even squares. Lastly, slice the squares down the diagonal to create 16 large triangles. If you want to create smaller scones, simply cut on the opposite diagonal to produce 32 smaller triangle scones.
- Transfer the scones to the prepared baking sheets with room to spread and bake for 20 minutes or until golden brown and desired texture is achieved.
- Let cool slightly before drizzling with the maple glaze.

WHILE THE SCONES ARE BAKING, MAKE THE MAPLE GLAZE

In a small saucepan over medium heat, begin melting the butter. Add the brown sugar and whisk until fully dissolved. Then, add the heavy cream and stir for another 2-3 minutes. Lastly, add the powdered sugar and continue to whisk until all the lumps have been incorporated. Turn the stove off and let it cool slightly before drizzling over cookies. Careful not to let the glaze harden before drizzling.

☆☆☆☆☆

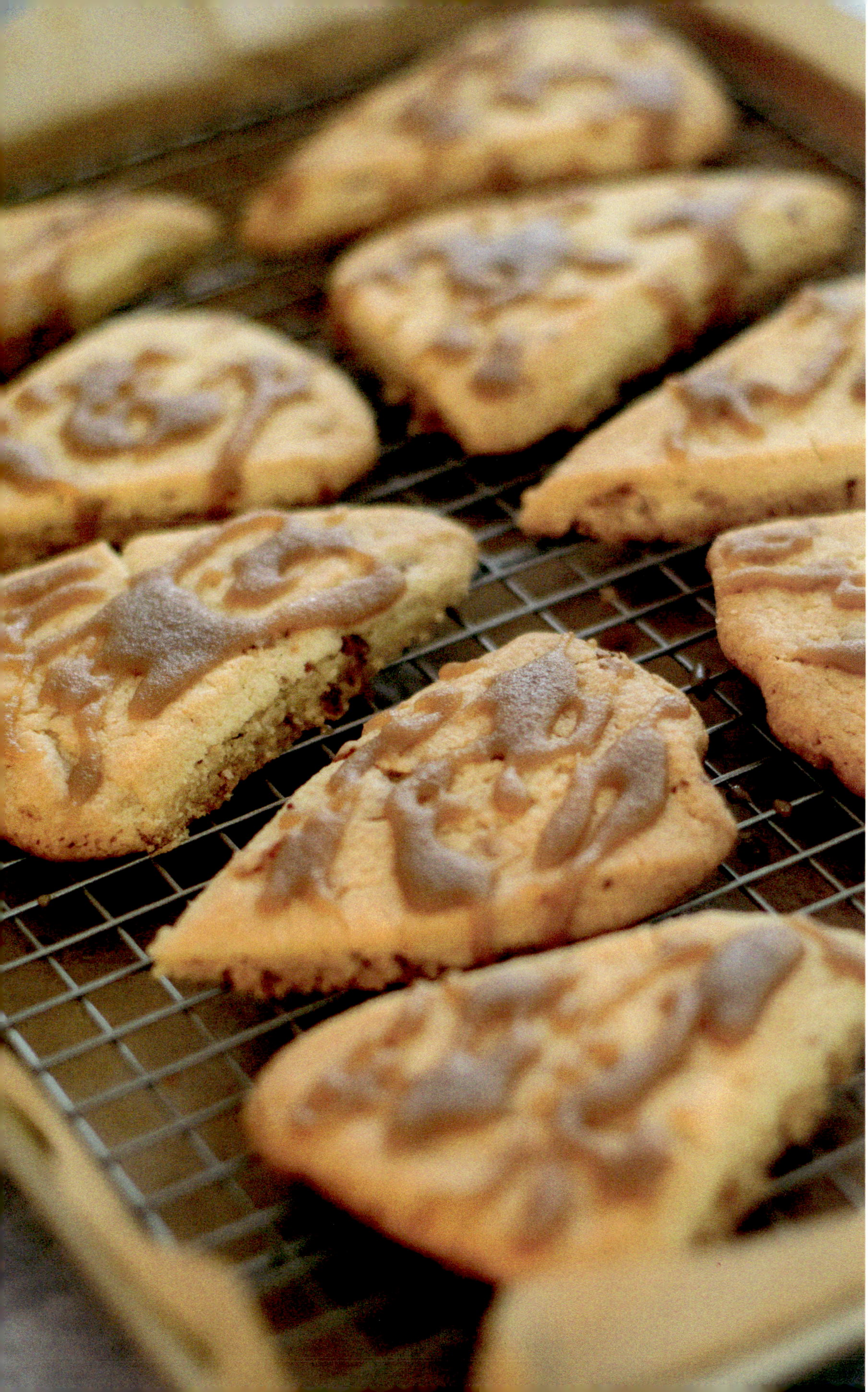

Egg Free

Nut Free

Soy Free

Pumpkin Pecan Quick Bread

The pumpkin baking season is a short one, it's long-awaited during the year, but once the clock strikes December, we seem to forget all about the wonders of "Fall Baking." The combination of hot, sweet bread baking in the oven and the smell of pumpkin spice filling the air is enough to make anybody happy while welcoming fall with open arms. This Pumpkin Pecan Bread is perfect for a chilly morning breakfast with a cup of hot coffee or even munch on for dessert after a warm bowl full of chili.

PREP TIME: 20 minutes

COOK TIME: 60 minutes

YIELDS: 1 Loaf (6-8 serving slices)

Ingredients:

1 ¾ cup all purpose flour

1 tsp baking soda

1 tsp baking powder

2 tsp pumpkin pie spice

¼ tsp salt

¼ cup liquid/melted coconut oil (or canola oil)

½ cup unsweetened applesauce

1 cup packed light brown sugar

1 large egg

1 cup pumpkin puree

1 tsp pure vanilla extract

½ cup semi-sweet chocolate chips

½ cup pecans, chopped

Directions:

- Preheat the oven to 350 degrees Fahrenheit. Prepare a single bread loaf pan with oil or butter and parchment paper- set aside for later.
- In a medium-sized mixing bowl, whisk together the flour, baking soda, baking powder, pumpkin pie spice, and salt. Set aside for later.
- In an electric mixer, combine the melted coconut oil, apple sauce, and packed brown sugar together on low for about 1 minute.
- Add the egg, pumpkin puree, and vanilla extract to the electric mixer and continue to mix on low for another 2-3 minutes.
- Slowly add the dry mixture (1 heaping spoonful at a time) to the mixer and continue to mix on low until all the flour is combined. Periodically scrape the bottom of the mixer to incorporate any loose flour.
- Add the chocolate chips to the batter and fold them in with a spatula. Pour the batter into the prepared bread loaf pan, spreading/leveling it out with a spatula.
- Sprinkle the chopped pecans on top and place in the oven to bake for 40 minutes.
- After 40 minutes, place a sheet of aluminum foil on top to prevent the pecans from burning. Bake for another 20 minutes (for a total of 60 minutes). Poke a toothpick in the center of the bread to determine when done.

Tips:

Can be stored at room temperature or in the refrigerator with aluminum foil or plastic wrap to cover the top.

Serve warm with a cup of hot coffee in the mornings, a cold glass of milk in the evenings, or try spreading some creamy almond butter over a slice for a midday snack.

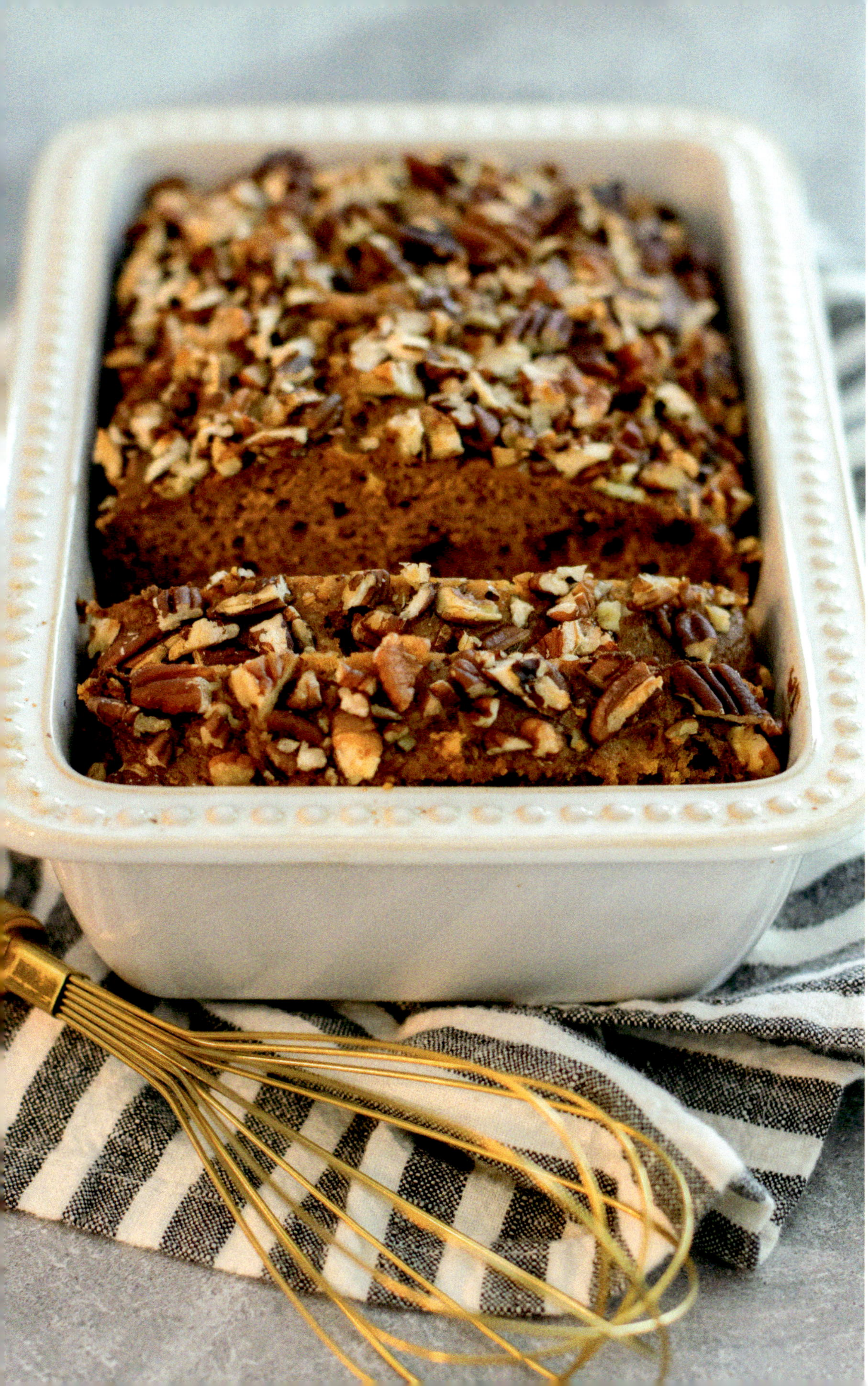

Dairy Free

Soy Free

Sweet & Salty Candied Pecans

These pecans have been a family Christmas tradition for the last several years. A few years back, I made this recipe for my family, and my brother immediately took an extreme liking to them. Not joking; he may have eaten all four cups of pecans himself. Since then, I make it a point to whip this recipe up for him (and the rest of my family, of course) every Christmas season. It's always special when you can gift a recipe to somebody who will appreciate it, especially around the holidays. These pecans make excellent gifts considering they travel well, don't need to be refrigerated, and there are endless wrapping options. Furthermore, I love that this recipe calls for egg whites instead of butter, reducing the calorie content and preventing the pecans from burning while baking for such a long time.

PREP TIME: 10 minutes

COOK TIME: 50 minutes

YIELDS: 4 cups of Pecans

Ingredients:

2 large egg whites

1 Tbsp water

4 cup pecans

1 cup granulated sugar

2 tsp coarse kosher salt

2 tsp ground cinnamon

Tip:

Can be stored at room temperature with aluminum foil or plastic wrap to cover the top.

Directions:

- Preheat the oven to 300 degrees Fahrenheit. Prepare a large baking sheet with parchment paper.
- In a large mixing bowl, whisk together the egg whites and water until the mixture becomes slightly foamy.
- Add the pecans into the egg white mixture. Using a spatula, mix until the pecans are evenly coated.
- In a small mixing bowl, whisk together the sugar, salt, and ground cinnamon. Pour the sugar coating on top of the pecans and continue to mix with the spatula until evenly coated.
- Pour the sugar-coated pecans on the prepared baking sheet, spreading them out to prevent excessive overlapping. Place in the oven for 25 minutes.
- After 25 minutes of the pecans baking, use a large, durable spatula to mix the pecans around the pan without taking them out of the oven. This helps to prevent them from sticking.
- Continue to bake the pecans for another 25 minutes.
- After a total bake time of 50 minutes, take the pecans out of the oven and immediately mix them around the parchment paper with the spatula to loosen/break up any pecans that may be sticking to the parchment paper. This step is essential in preventing the pecans from sticking to or tearing the parchment paper. Let cool completely before transferring the pecans to a separate serving dish.

☆☆☆☆☆

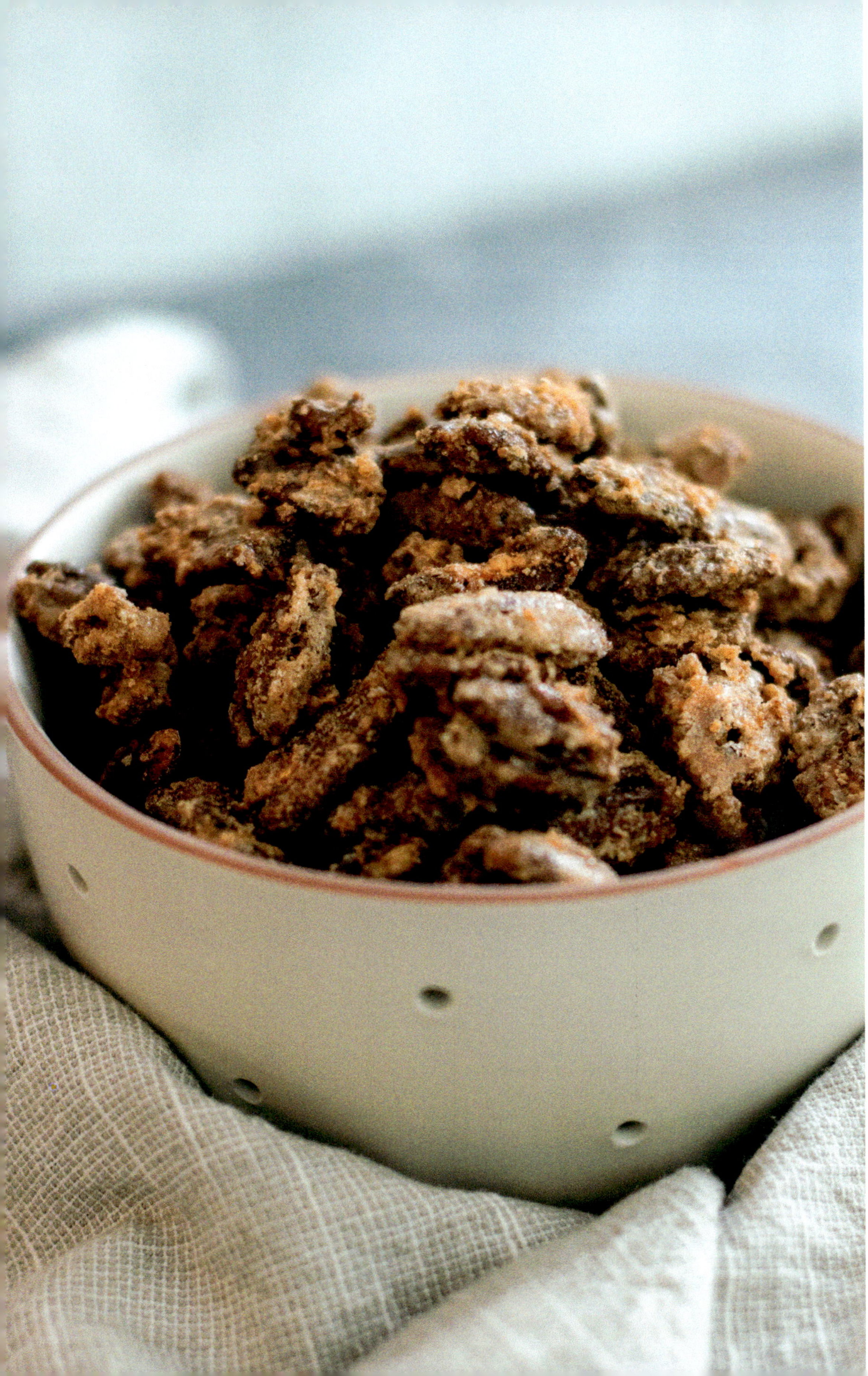

Gluten Free

Dairy Free

Soy Free

My Infamous Traditional Cinnamon Rolls

Forever stamped as our family's favorite indulgent breakfast, these cinnamon rolls go down in history as the best (yet most time-consuming) recipe in this entire cookbook. Traditionally, I only make these cinnamon rolls on Christmas morning and occasionally throughout the year for big celebrations because of the time it takes from start to finish. I first made these cinnamon rolls the weekend after Justin and I got married. We had been going non-stop for months with appointments, to-do lists, itineraries, and meetings. All we desperately wanted was a lazy weekend together paired with a phenomenal breakfast. I think I earned the "best wife" status that weekend when I whipped these cinnamon rolls up from scratch. Since then, the recipe has changed only slightly, modifying only what's necessary while keeping the gooey, decadent taste present. These simple yet incredibly sweet rolls are perfect for celebrating birthday mornings, anniversaries, or any other special occasion in between.

PREP TIME: 40 minutes

INACTIVE RISE TIME: 2 hours

COOK TIME: 20-24 minutes

YIELDS: 110 large cinnamon rolls

Ingredients:

1 small package (¼ oz) active dry yeast

1 cup warm milk

½ cup granulated sugar

⅓ cup butter, softened

½ tsp salt

2 large eggs

4 cups all purpose flour

1 cup packed light brown sugar

3 tbsp ground cinnamon

⅓ cup butter, softened

6 tbsp butter, softened

1 ½ cup confectioner's sugar

⅓ cup Philadelphia cream cheese, softened

½ tsp pure vanilla extract

Tip:

Can be stored in the refrigerator in the same container they were baked in for up to 7 days. Place aluminum foil or plastic wrap over the top while storing.

Directions:

- In a measuring cup or small bowl, dissolve the yeast in the warm milk. Gently whisk together to help incorporate the yeast granules but do not overmix. (make sure the milk is not hot as this will harm the yeast and thereby preventing the dough from rising)
- Using an electric mixer fitted with a dough paddle and a large mixing bowl, add the sugar, butter, salt, eggs, and flour. Mix until incorporated. Add the yeast mixture and continue to mix until dough is formed.
- Cover and let rise for 1-2 hours in a warm place or until the dough has risen (does not have to double in size).
- After the dough has risen, preheat the oven to 350 degrees Fahrenheit and grease the bottom of a 9x13 inch baking dish. Roll the dough onto a lightly floured surface, resembling more of a long rectangle instead of a circle.
- Rinse the mixing bowl and prepare to use it again for the cinnamon filling. Using the whisk attachment, mix together the brown sugar, cinnamon, and ⅓ cup of softened butter until crumbly. Spread the cinnamon mixture evenly over the rolled-out dough, making sure to reach all the way to the edges. The cinnamon mixture is tough to work with if using a spatula; I recommend using your hands to work it into the dough.
- Begin rolling up the dough like a sleeping bag, starting from the longest side, not the short side. Slice into 1 ½ inch rolls. Place in the prepared pan and let rise for another 30 minutes to 1 hour until they have risen again and increased in size.
- Bake for 20-24 minutes. While the rolls are baking, begin making the cream cheese icing. Using the electric mixer and rinsed mixing bowl, combine and mix the 6 tbsp butter, powdered sugar, cream cheese, and vanilla until smooth and creamy.
- Cinnamon rolls are done baking when the centers are slightly firm to the touch and edges are slightly golden. Do not overbake. When the rolls are done baking, let cool slightly before spreading icing over the cinnamon rolls.

☆☆☆☆☆

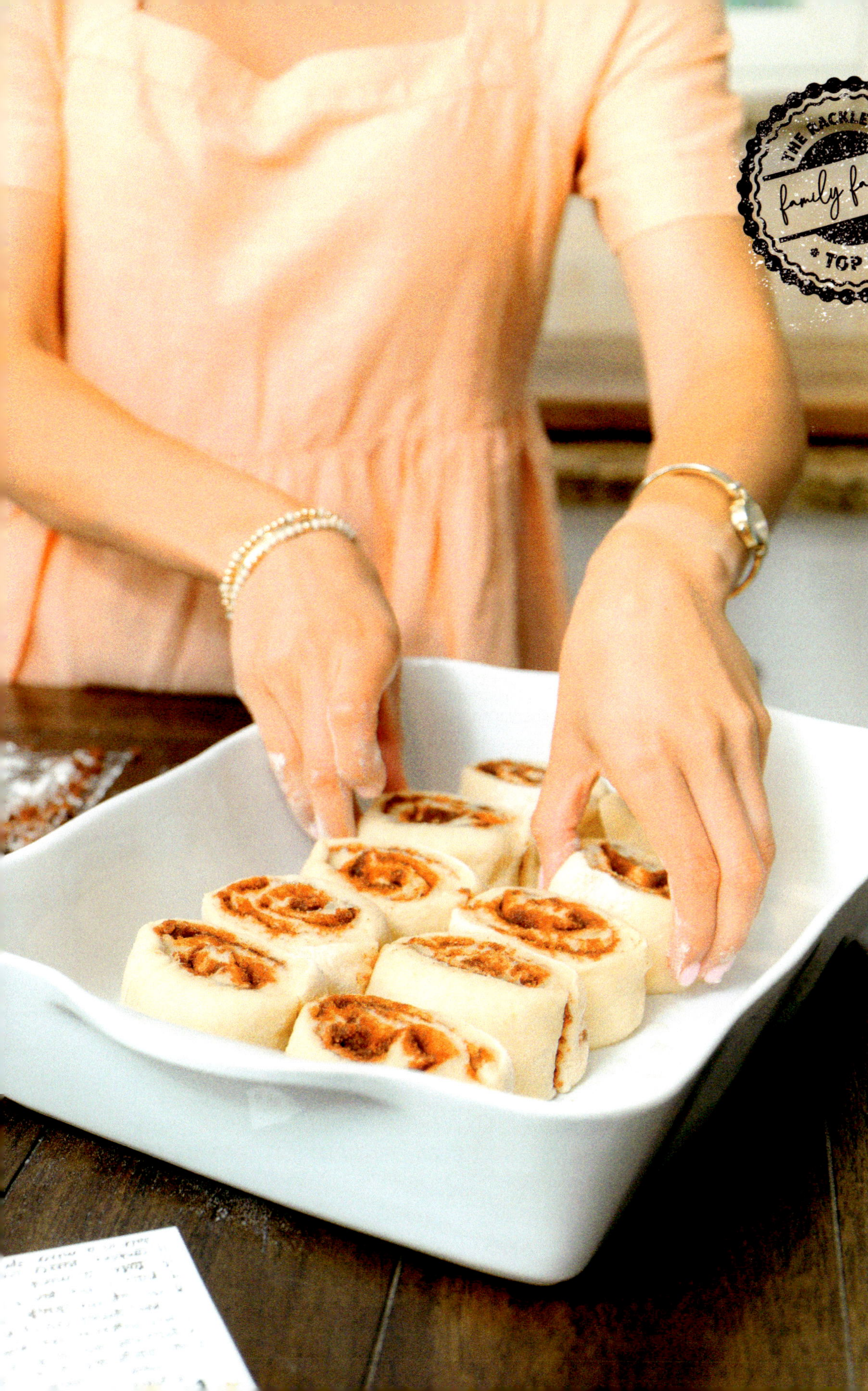

Nut Free

Soy Free

Life's Peachy & Crisp

Life's full of peachy moments, like when you whip up a homemade dessert in 15 minutes, and it tastes like it could win a gold medal at a local pie contest. Although not quite considered a pie or cobbler, a crisp is determined by the streusel-like topping consisting of oats and good old-fashioned flour. This dessert is a favorite of ours during the summertime when the peaches are ripe, and the vanilla ice cream is plentiful. Although you can make this crisp dish year-round because it requires only frozen peaches, just don't tell anybody your secret for deliciousness.

PREP TIME: 15 minutes

COOK TIME: 45-50 minutes

YIELDS: (1) 9" Pie

Ingredients:

1 (1lb) bag frozen sliced peaches

½ cup granulated sugar

1 tsp ground cinnamon

2 tsp cornstarch

1 cup all purpose flour

8 tbsp cold salted butter,
cut into tbsp pats

½ cup old fashioned rolled oats

2 tbsp pure maple syrup

½ cup granulated sugar

Directions:

- Preheat the oven to 375 degrees Fahrenheit. Prepare a 9" pie dish with a light layer of cooking spray.
- In a mixing bowl, add the peaches, sugar, cinnamon, and cornstarch. Using a rubber spatula, mix to combine and pour contents into the prepared baking pie dish. -In a separate mixing bowl, whisk together the flour and sugar. Using a pastry cutter, begin cutting the cold butter into the flour mixture until it resembles coarse crumbs
- Add the rolled oats and maple syrup and continue to incorporate together using a rubber spatula.
- Pour the flour mixture on top of the peaches and spread evenly, reaching the edges of the pie dish.
- Place the pie dish on a large baking sheet (to prevent drippings onto the oven bottom) and bake for 45-50 minutes or until the peach filling begins to bubble and the crisp topping begins to brown slightly.
- Let cool completely before serving to prevent the peach filling from spilling out.

Tips:

Store in the refrigerator with aluminum foil or plastic wrap on top for up to 1 week. Perfect to serve with vanilla ice cream or a cold glass of milk.

☆☆☆☆☆

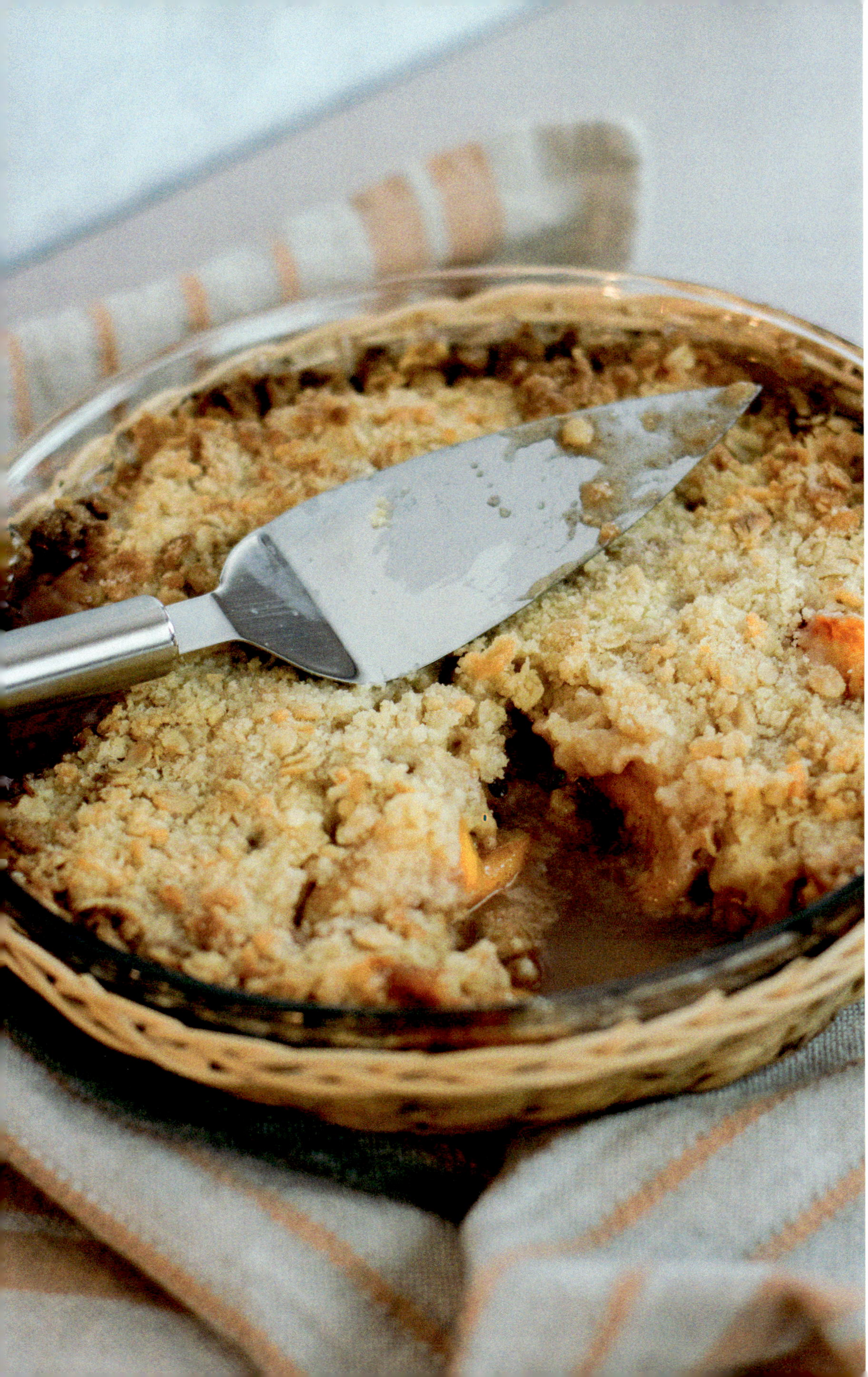

Nut Free

Egg Free

Soy Free

Simple Strawberry Rhubarb Jam

This homemade jam recipe is such a great way to get kids involved in the kitchen. I recommend having everything pre-chopped, sliced, and zested before the children join you. I've even prepped the fruit the night before and made jam the following day. Once prepped, this recipe is easy enough for kids to help without too many steps to overwhelm them. Just make sure you take the ropes on the canning part. The bonus is getting to celebrate at the end with a homemade peanut butter and jelly sandwich like no other. Not only does this recipe make quite a few mason jars of homemade jam for future use, but the jam-filled jars also make perfect gifts for any occasion.

A tip for extra added fun: If you live near a pick-it-yourself strawberry farm, go pick the strawberries first and make your own jam. The taste of homemade, homegrown strawberry jam is truly unmatched. And of course, my absolute favorite way to enjoy homemade jam is smothered on freshly baked buttermilk biscuits in the morning.

PREP TIME: 30 minutes

CANNING & COOLING TIME: 1 hour

COOK TIME: 1 hour

YIELDS: 8-10 (8 oz) mason jars

Ingredients:

4 ½ - 5 cups diced fresh strawberries

4 cups diced fresh rhubarb (about 4-5 large stalks)

2 (1.75 oz) packages powdered fruit pectin. (Can be found in the Jell-O or mason jar section of the store)

2 tbsp butter, cold

1 large orange (zested and juiced)

4-5 cups granulated sugar

Tips:

Unopened, properly sealed jars can be stored at room temperature for up to 1 year.

Once opened, store in the refrigerator for up to 2 months.

Directions:

MAKING THE JAM

- Wash and dry 8-10 8oz mason jars with new lids.
- Wash all produce before preparation. Cut away any tough, woody, or bruised parts of the rhubarb stalks and peel away the red flesh (like you would with celery stalks). This gives way to a green rhubarb stalk. Dice the prepped rhubarb and strawberries into small pieces.
- In a large stockpot over medium heat, add the diced strawberries, diced rhubarb, both packages of pectin, butter, orange zest, and orange juice. Mix to combine and bring to a soft bubble to condense down, occasionally stirring to prevent sticking/burning.
- Once the fruit is condensed down quite a bit (about 30-45 minutes of bubbling), add the sugar, 1 cup at a time until fully dissolved. Continue to stir to prevent foaming on top.
- Once the sugar is dissolved and the jam consistency is to your liking (I prefer very small chunks of fruit), bring the heat up to a full boil. Let the jam boil for 1-2 minutes.
- Turn the stove off and let the jam rest for about 10 minutes. If there is any foam, simply remove this by scraping it with a spoon or spatula.
- Using a jar funnel, pour the jam into each mason jar with about 1/2 inch remaining at the top. Cover tightly with the appropriate pre-washed mason jar lids.

CANNING PROCESS

- Place the jelly-filled mason jars in a clean, large stockpot. Fill the stockpot with water until the jars are completely submerged. Place the stockpot on the stove over high heat and bring it to a boil. Let it continue to boil for 8-10 minutes.
- Once the jars have sealed, turn the stove off and let the water cool off quite a bit before attempting to take the jars out. Using large tongs or grabbers, carefully take the jars out of the hot water bath and place them on a cooling rack to set. The jars will be sealed completely when cooled and punched down; this typically takes about 30-60 minutes of cooling.

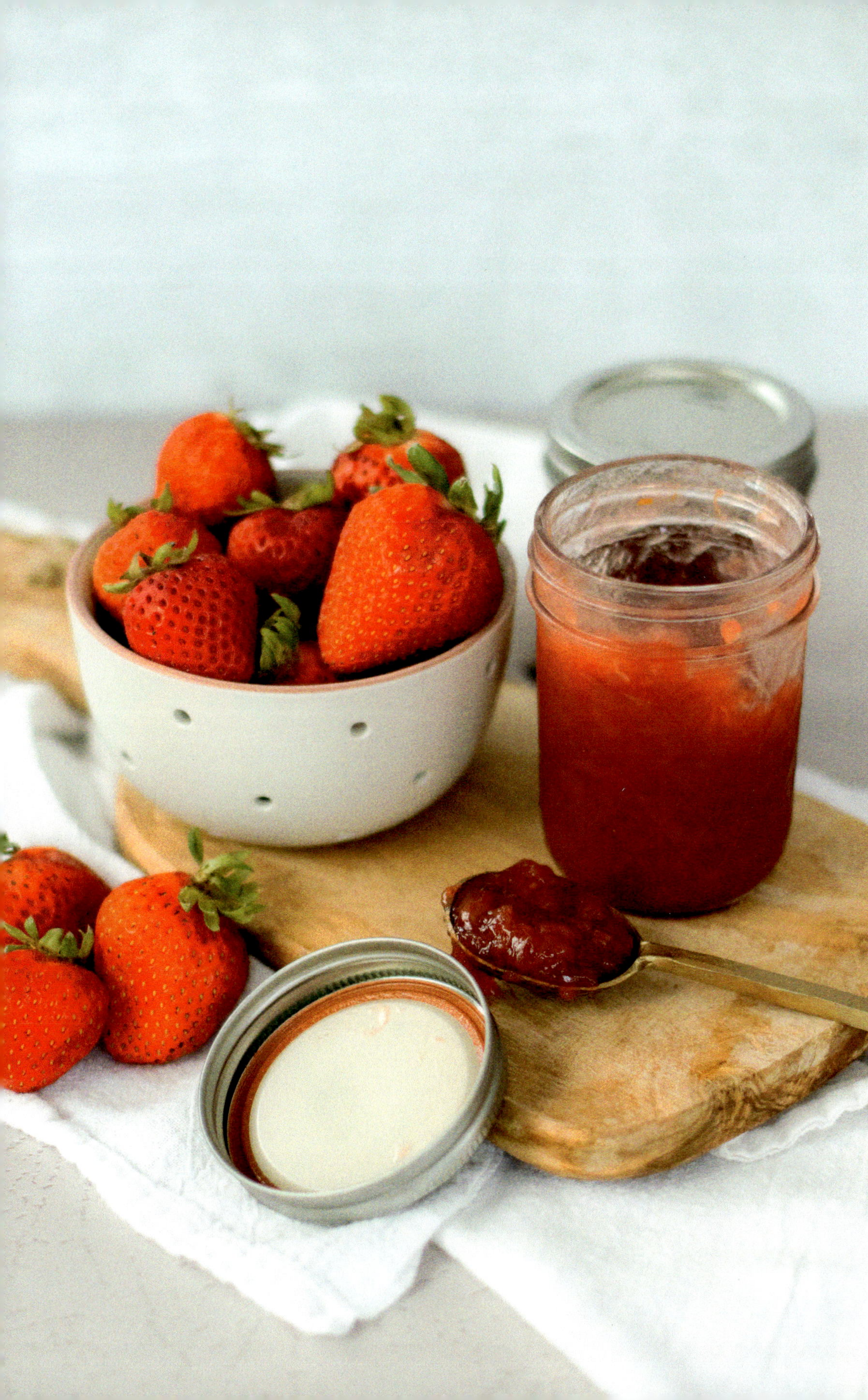

Gluten Free

Egg Free

Nut Free

Soy Free

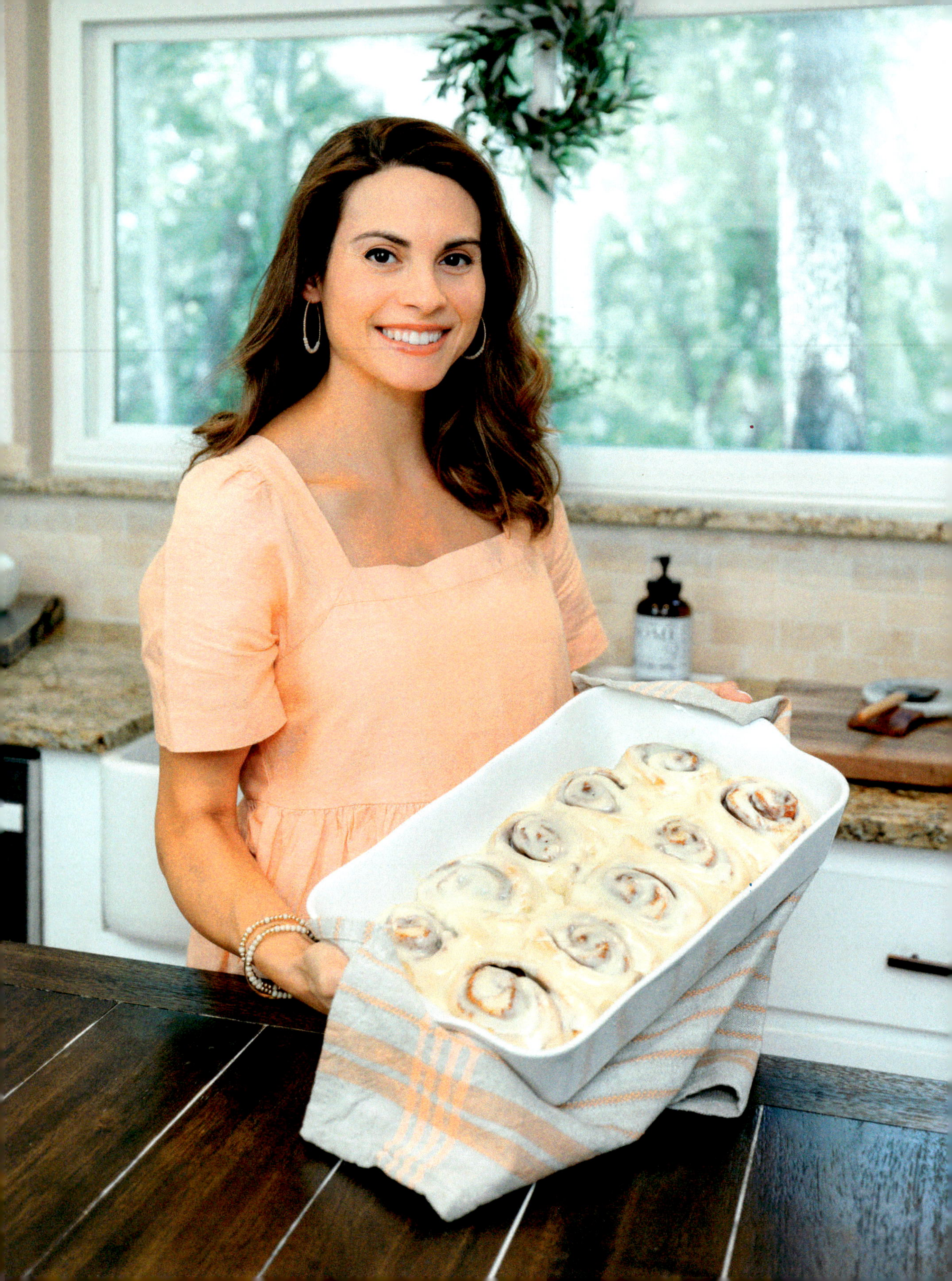

About the Author

Stephanie Rackley is a Registered and Licensed Dietitian practicing in the Texas DFW area. She was a Kilgore College Rangerette in 2011-2013, to whom she owes her discipline, positive outlook, and determination. She graduated from Texas A&M University with a bachelor's degree in Nutritional Science and completed her Dietetic Internship shortly afterward. After gaining her credentials, she created 'The Healthy Chew' blog and social platform in 2015 with the intention of spreading helpful nutrition knowledge and healthy recipes to her followers. She then created a private consulting business, 'AVO Good Life Nutrition LLC' for individuals struggling with nutrition and food choices. Stephanie has been interviewed and featured in VoyageDallas as part of their local entrepreneur series and has collaborated with renowned brands like Bertolli®, CVS Health®, Vital Proteins®, and HelloFresh®. Although she loved nutrition consulting one-on-one with the clients she met and helped, her daughter, Emery, took priority once she was born.

Today, The Healthy Chew has become a more prominent brand that encompasses whole family health, weekly meal recipe ideas, and aims to promote body and overall life positivity. Since having her first child- Emmie, Stephanie has shifted her focus to raising her family at home. She and her husband, Justin, share their love for the outdoors while raising Emmie. They have showcased their honest outdoor lifestyle on YouTube as part of their channel, Lake Life Family. Furthermore, Stephanie is known for always cooking or baking something from scratch, whether it be wild game meats, homemade desserts, or anything in-between. Stephanie and Justin will soon welcome their second child, Benjamin River.

References

- Brazier, Yvette. "The Health Benefits of Almonds." ***Medical News Today***, 12 Dec. 2019, www.medicalnewstoday.com/articles/269468.

  ---. "What Are the Health Benefits of Oregano?" Medical News Today, 17 Jan. 2020, www.medicalnewstoday.com/articles/266259.

  ---. "What to Know about Apples." Medical News Today, 18 Dec. 2019, www.medicalnewstoday.com/articles/267290.
- Foret, Rosalee de la. ***Alchemy of Herbs.*** New York, United States, Penguin Random House, 2017.
- Grotto, David, and Lisa Lillien. ***The Best Things You Can Eat.*** Hachette Book Group, 2013.
- Horton, Brierley M. "The Amazing Health Benefits of Zucchini." ***EatingWell,*** 22 July 2021, www.eatingwell.com/article/7805709/the-amazing-health-benefits-of-zucchini.
- Leonard, Jayne. "What Are the Benefits of Pistachios?" ***Medical News Today,*** 29 Aug. 2018, www.medicalnewstoday.com/articles/322899.
- Petre, Alina M. "How Chai Tea Can Improve Your Health." ***Healthline***, 20 July 2017, www.healthline.com/nutrition/chai-tea.
- Sorrells, Ally. "Amazing Health Benefits of Peaches." ***EatingWell***, 23 Jan. 2021, www.eatingwell.com/article/292214/amazing-health-benefits-of-peaches.
- Ware, Megan. "Benefits and Health Risks of Bananas." ***Medical News Today,*** 13 Jan. 2020, www.medicalnewstoday.com/articles/271157.

  ---. "Everything You Need to Know about Blueberries." ***Medical News Today,*** 5 Sept. 2017, www.medicalnewstoday.com/articles/287710.

  ---. "What Are the Health Benefits of Chives?" ***Medical News Today***, 27 Jan. 2020, www.medicalnewstoday.com/articles/275009.
- West, Helen R. "6 Evidence-Based Health Benefits of Lemons." ***Healthline,*** 7 Jan. 2019, www.healthline.com/nutrition/6-lemon-health-benefits.
- Zemser, Rachel. "To Understand Walnut Flavor, Get Under the Skin -."***California Walnuts,*** 28 Oct. 2013, walnuts.org/news/to-understand-walnut-flavor-get-under-the-skin-california-walnuts.

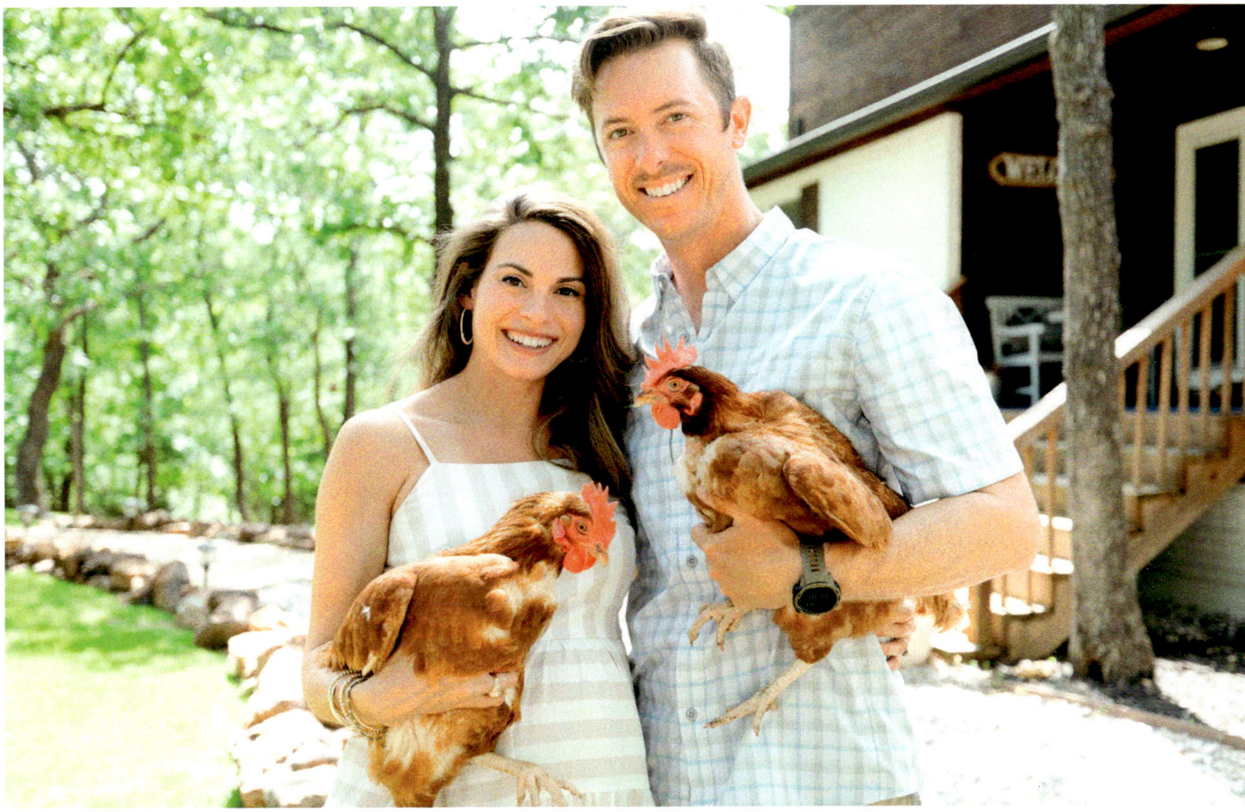

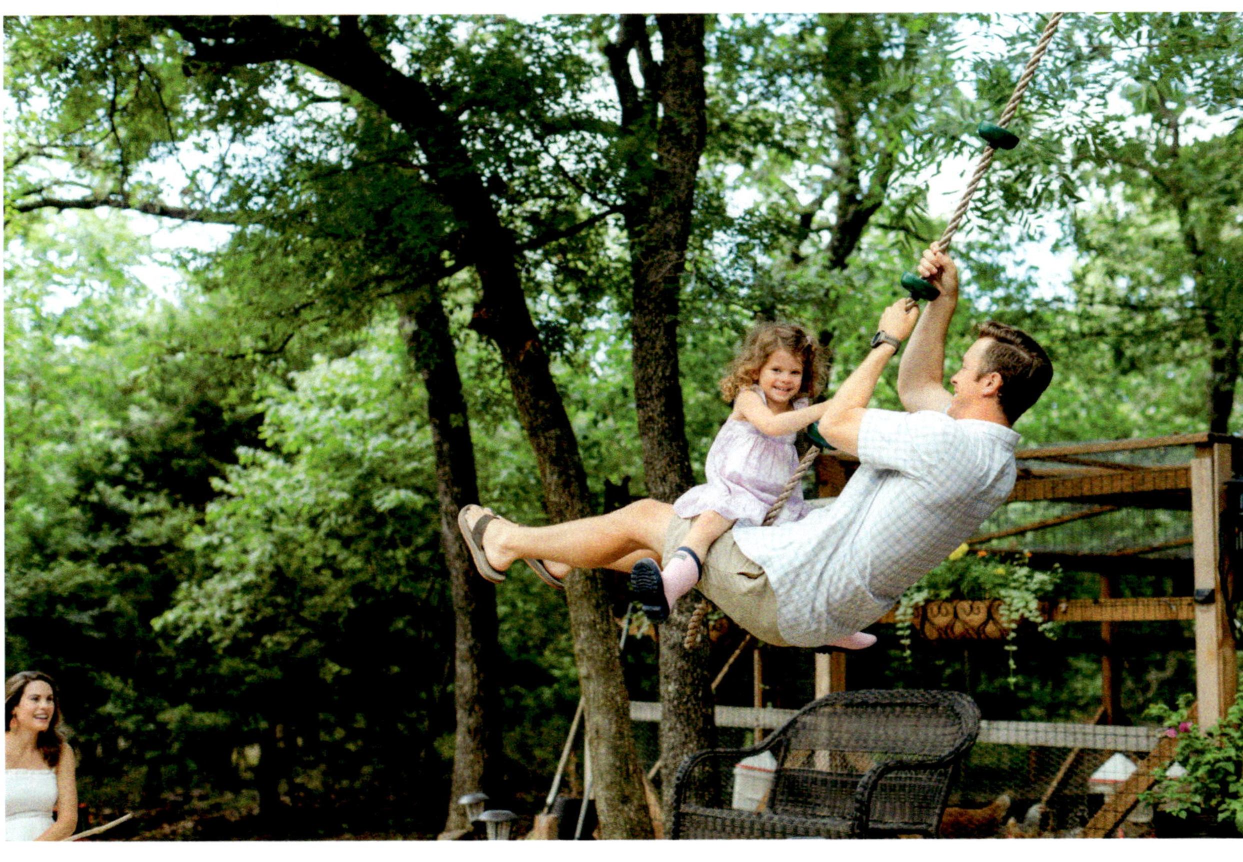

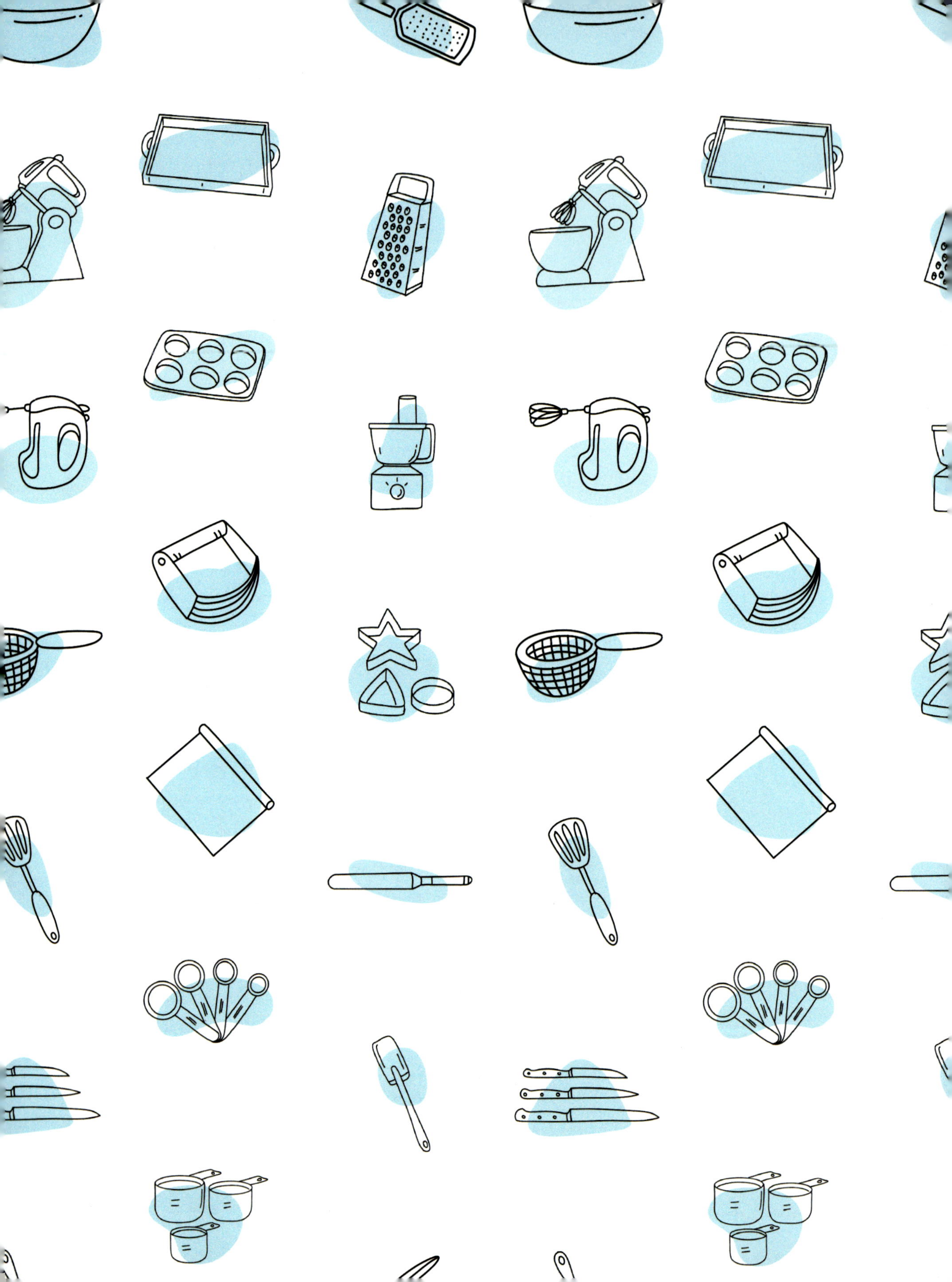